I Am A Beautiful

FLOWER

WHAT EVERY FLOWERING GIRL SHOULD KNOW

MARLO Y. ETTIEN

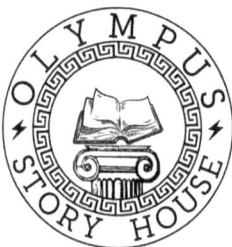

Olumpus Story House
www.olympusstoryhouse.com

CONTENTS

Introduction 1

A Word from the Doctor 8

Basic Biology: The Cycle Begins 10

Reproductive System Vocabulary 22

Nutrition for a Healthy Reproductive System 46

Water 48

Vitamins 50

The 21 Essential Minerals Your Mind and Body Needs 59

Electrolytes 71

Amino Acids 76

Herbal Support for the Reproductive
and Immune Systems 86

What Are Digestive Enzymes? 102

Prebiotics vs. Probiotics 105

Pregnancy 110

Pregnancy Month to Month 113

Will the Fetus be Female or Male?

What Determines the Sex? 126

References 131

Glossary 136

Appendixes 175

Conclusion 187

"This beautiful book will help daughters AND mothers. It shows how fellowship can heal the past and make the future healthy. It shows women working together (in a way against the prevailing culture) to restore dignity and improve life for everybody. Congratulations on a wonderful, useful, healing book."

Dr. Barbara D. Massey
Associate Professor of Philosophy and Religion
Emerita Chatham University

"From the very beginning, the book is captivating! It pulls you in and takes you to a place of love and peace through the normal process of the human body. What a beautiful gift Ettien has given to her daughter (and mothers and daughters everywhere), who has made and are making the transition from childhood into womanhood. Through the sharing of this experience together, they will always be connected by this "miracle moment." The perfect book for mother and daughter."

Pamela Tate
Author/Mentor

"A much needed and refreshing work that is appropriate for many cultures and those of various religions.

Written in a tone that is matter-of-fact and never condescending or infantilizing. Provides emotional support and comfort. While the title suggests that its primary audience is girls, it actually has a much broader audience of men, women, and boys, who know and love girls. Boys, girls, women and men need and deserve to know the information contained in this work.

Contains clear, easy to comprehend biological explanations of menstruation, ovulation, fertilization and pregnancy, as well as male anatomy and experiences. Provides selected vocabulary, as well as nicknames or slang terms to help the uninitiated and those who must cross generation gaps or divides.

Several captivating pieces of information are included throughout the work. "Only elephants, humpback whales and human females undergo menopause."

There is a wealth of practical information about the discomforts associated with menstruation and a description of a wide range of remedies. The suggestions for how to handle menstrual flow help to debunk many myths. The nutrition and hydration information and suggestions are invaluable. Useful references for further exploration are provided."

Dr. Karen Dajani-Rochez
Professor Emeritus, Communications Department
Chatham University

Banvoa's Journey

When I think of Africa,

and envision the continent,
I see through the rough terrain,
the eyes, nose and mouth of
a girl child, especially her eyes.
They are longing for freedom,
intense with readiness,
and gentle with hope.

Marlo Y. Ettien

Acknowledgements

We give thanks for motherhood and awareness of how to guide Banvoa regarding her body, celebrating her into womanhood. We give thanks to all the women who created a sacred circle of wisdom in support of Banvoa during her Flowering Party and Promise Ring Gathering (Tiara, Barbara, Malane, Ursula, Rickenya, Toni, Robin, Linda, Gwennie, Karen, Antoinette, Sandra, Gloria, Sharron, Ayanna, Marva, Madina, and Geri.)

We thank Emmanuel Adouobo for his fond admiration of his sister.

Now to Armel N'Guessan Ettien, Banvoa Sudarkasa Ettien's Daddy, the first man in her life, who named her. Thank you for covering our daughter Banvoa with your love, honoring her with your presence, guiding her with your wisdom, instructing her with your intelligence, and protecting her with your prayers and resolve.

We give thanks to all people working to help developing children better understanding their bodies, as part of their sacred circle, whether they are aware of it or not.

Dedication

To all the girls around the world, you are a beautiful flower, a lotus. And your body, your life is sacred. I cherish you.

Lotuses are symbols of purity, divine birth and beauty, an exquisite flower. Lotus is regarded as the perfect and divine flower symbolizing beauty and spirituality in several different cultures and religions of the world. The lotus grows in the muddy water of still ponds and lakes. The magnificent blossom unfolds gradually, one petal at a time, till full bloom in the morning when the sun's rays touch the flower. As the lotus awakens and blooms at the first rays of the morning sun, the interdependence between the lotus and the sun is a symbol of love.

The pink lotus is the supreme lotus and is considered sacred.

If stories come to you, care for them.
And learn to give them away where they are needed. Sometimes a person needs a story
more than food to stay alive.

Barry Lopez

Introduction

The menstrual cycle phases are a powerful, intimate time for females. It is a time of the month that is uniquely different for all females, as each female's body is different. It should be an honored time treated as sacred and, most of all, celebrated. No girl should fear her menstrual cycle or be embarrassed because of experiencing it from month to month. Rather, she should be aware and empowered with knowledge and comforted through support. Every month, there are a certain number of fertile days in which a healthy female who has started her menstrual cycle can become pregnant. Every developing girl needs to know her days and that these fertility days can vary monthly. Each girl should be guided to learn to cherish herself and avoid giving away the sacredness of her sexual power that may result in an unwanted pregnancy. In having a basic understanding of the biology of their bodies, perhaps fewer teen girls will become pregnant.

Although some girls reading this book may not have a close relationship with their mothers (or fathers who may be more involved in the girl's life as a caregiver), perhaps this book will offer the treasured validation they need to know that they are loved. Please remember beautiful flowers, you are surrounded by love–a love that is trustworthy and nurturing. You need only acknowledge it in the women reaching out to you, offering their mothering and guidance along your life's journey. Please accept it. This book is written for you as a keepsake to provide some basic loving information about the reproductive system.

Thus, the idea for this book begins with my own story–a story of welcoming my daughter, Banvoa, into womanhood with love and celebration rather than fear and uncertainty. It is a story for which I as a mother; continue to offer guidance to my daughter deeply rooted in respect and responsibility. A story about strengthening a common bond of interconnectedness from one generation to the next–an empowering bond that is nurturing in its mindfulness of how sacred the female body is in its ability to carry life.

Since infancy, I had been sharing with Banvoa how to care for her body. It has been my intention to teach her to be confident and comfortable with herself as a female. So, I began telling her the exact names of her parts, such as vagina, rather than "tee tee." When she was three, I began to teach her about personal space and where she should not be touched. As an inquisitive five-year-old who asked, "Where do babies come from?" I explained that Mommy and Daddy helped to create her, how I carried her in my stomach and pointed to my navel and hers to show where we had been connected. It was then that I bought the DVD—"NOVA: The Miracle of Life" for us to watch together. When she turned 10, we talked again about personal space and boys. This was when I had begun to anticipate Banvoa's period and prepare myself mentally and emotionally as her breast began to develop—praying that it would not happen now. Yet knowing when it did happen, I wanted to be ready to help her understand its importance.

A few months before Banvoa turned 12 on March 29, 2009, she began complaining about headaches and taking more naps. Since there were no other symptoms to think it was a cold or virus, I thought it might be her period. I began to think about a care kit for her locker, the pads she would use, if she wanted to use pads or tampons, would she start it at home or school. I had preferred it to be at home so I would be there for her, helping her know what to do.

On Wednesday, March 23, a few days before her birthday, during a tutoring session with three of her neighborhood friends, who are also sisters, Banvoa stood from the dining table. Because of the look of discomfort on her face, I asked, "What's the matter? Why are you standing?"

" In a soft low voice, she replied, "My stomach hurts."

Ever ready to soothe a pain, I asked, "Where does it hurt?"

Banvoa said, "Down there." "Your abdomen?

"Yes."

I paused momentarily, feeling sure and joyful about what it could be, in a playful singing voice, I said, "Banvoa, it's your period." She looked a little fearful and unsure. It was quiet for a moment, as her father and brother stopped eating and turned to look at her. While the three sisters turned to each other, seemingly silently reminiscing over the common bond they already shared, perhaps remembering when they each started. Noticing Banvoa's fear, I knew it was time to share my period story to console her. I was ready and happy to share a treasured part of myself that was a positive exchange between my mother, grandmother, and me.

I told them when I was 13 years-old, playing at Frick Park (in Pittsburgh, PA), I took a break from playing to use the restroom and noticed a blood stain on my panties—I began to search my legs for a cut, not knowing what was happening. I left the park wondering how I could be bleeding without a wound. I went to my grandmother's house to tell my mother what happened. As I sat on the living room couch, my mother went into the kitchen to talk with my grandmother. Grandma Lil called me into the kitchen. I knew it was important since the kitchen table seemed to be the place to share all important news. After I sat down, Grandma Lil with a deep sense of knowing on her face, bent over to meet my face and with a smile told me, "You're a woman now. You can have babies."

My mother said, "You started your period." They explained what I needed to do to care for my body. While my mother and grandmother discussed how much money would be needed to buy pads, I went back to the living room couch to consider this new person I had become. I was mystified by what it meant to be a mother, considering how I never really thought about it—did not need to think about it until then. At that moment, I began thinking differently about my body.

After I finished my story, the sisters one by one, were glad to share theirs. After the girls finished their stories, Banvoa continued her session. I looked over at my husband and son, who silently listened with blank stares, unsure if they should feel uncomfortable or privileged to witness the wonderment of intergenerational female bonding. With Banvoa now at ease, glowing from the comforting warmth of our stories, I began to think about what more I could do to help her to know that her period should be embraced not feared. Although I had been discussing her transition into womanhood for years, including the difference between being a teen mother in America and a married mother, I wanted her experience to be more empowering than mine to carry on a tradition of female bonding and acceptance. I thought about having a party, all women, friends and family. The women with their wealth of experiences and understanding would offer Banvoa their comforting stories and gift baskets with things to pamper her during her special time of the month. It would be a celebration as she entered womanhood. I thought of the various herbal teas I drank over the years during my cycle, and the different books that I have read about the body. The stories I remembered about what other women from varying cultures do during their menses, separating themselves from their daily routine to pray, and sometimes fast, experiencing a more heightened intuitive awareness. Simply being more mindful of nurturing themselves, care for themselves, and loving themselves as women.

The next day, I shared my intentions with Armel and asked him to think of something he and Emmanuel could do together on the day of the party. I sent an e-mail to my women friends, making them aware of Banvoa's symptoms and the wonderful experience of sharing I had with the girls. I reminded them that her 12th birthday would be that Sunday and wanted to have a flowering party for her in April. The friends thought it was an interesting idea and were happy to participate. I asked them to offer her pampering gift baskets. I suggested herbal tea, toiletries, candles, and books, things I knew Banvoa would enjoy. I wanted to offer her something she would always cherish and remember, perhaps offer to her own daughter. I thought of adornments and bought Banvoa a beautiful butterfly necklace of yellow, white and rose gold. It was a perfect gift to symbolize her transformation.

As I prepared for the party, shopping for her gift and a book on the menstrual cycle, I met lovely people, some who gasped with joy about the flowering party and others who were fascinated with curiosity about what a flowering party is, since they had never heard of one. After I explained my intention, they thought it was a wonderful and intriguing idea. I will never forget the saleswoman who helped me pick Banvoa's necklace. We talked for about an hour. She was in her seventies and vividly remembered her own story and shared it with me. She blessed Banvoa with well wishes for her entry into womanhood. What was quite different were the responses of some of Banvoa's friends, who said, "Ewww." I took delight in explaining to the girls what their periods symbolizes and how it was not something to think about negatively.

The party was Saturday, April 25th, 2009 at 6. The women who could not attend the party that were out of state, sent their gifts by mail. One of my dearest friends, Gloria, whom I have known for more than 20 years, flew in from California to attend. Aunt Gloria helped create Banvoa's invitation. A young girl surrounded by a circle of women. The Kemetian (Egyptian) Mother Goddess Nut must have been ensuring that Banvoa's entry into womanhood would be memorable. The weekend before the party, Banvoa had the luxury of enjoying an all-girls pampering camp with one of her friends, who invited her.

On Friday evening before the party, Gloria, Tiara (cousin), Banvoa and me, went to Emory University to meet Alice Walker, who was being celebrated for her life's work. At the end of Ms. Walker's sharing aspects of her life's work, I had an opportunity to thank Ms. Walker for the impact her writing had on my life. I shared with the audience how as a youth, my Uncle Reggie gave me the "Color Purple" to read. I shared how the first research paper I had ever written in an English Literature class was on the women in her books, which I still have. I shared how Ms. Walker's books helped me celebrate myself as a woman, particularly a Black woman. And now being a mother, how I was teaching Banvoa to celebrate herself as a female. I was enormously proud to share with everyone that we were having a flowering party to celebrate Banvoa's entry into womanhood. The audience applauded and some even came to their feet to celebrate with us. It was a radiating honor filling us all with light.

The evening of the party, we ate and talked with Banvoa, at times individually, about her gifts as she opened them. For the friends who mailed their gifts, I read their cards and stories, sharing their gifts with Banvoa. The gifts were a treasure. Not only did Banvoa receive thoughtfully written cards, but she was also lavished with carefully prepared gift baskets, a precious scrapbook, a life-giving flower plant, wise personal stories, anchoring books, a loving spa treatment, and money to treat herself to whatever. After she opened all her gifts from her Aunties, I offered her my gift. I told her how much I loved her and was proud to offer her the necklace to symbolize the change she would experience.

She was so happy and grateful. Aunt Ursula shared with Banvoa that she was now a part of a circle of women who will always be available to her. We had an enlightening roundtable discussion at the kitchen table led by Aunt Gwennie, the elder in the group. It was real talk about virtuousness, morality, integrity, wisdom, intelligence, personal hygiene, entrepreneurship, spiritual and emotional strength, and men and boys. As we talked with Banvoa and as she listened, the contours of her beaming face softly revealed the comfort that was nurturing her.

The party was perfectly timed. Banvoa's first menstrual cycle started the next month on May 18th. This is her story...

On that unsuspecting day, Wednesday, May 20, 2009, at approximately 4:14 p.m., Emmanuel and I pulled into the driveway to meet Banvoa as she departed the school bus. It was a warm and sunny day. After putting our things inside the house, Emmanuel and I went back outside to the yard to play catch. The front door was open, and I heard, "Mom, Mom..."

I went just inside the door and asked, "Banvoa are you calling me?"

"Yes. Would you come here?"

So, I went to the powder room and opened the door. And she said, "Look." I said, "BANVOA, IT'S YOUR PERIOD! Let me go upstairs to get a pad and clean underwear."

I ran upstairs to get what she needed and ran back downstairs to the powder room and Emmanuel was outside the powder room door asking, "Banvoa, what's happening? What's going on?"

She calmly replied, "It's my period."

He said, "Oh."

I went inside the powder room and asked Banvoa to take off her panties and put on the clean ones. As she was sitting on the toilet, I gave her the pad and she asked, "Okay. What do I do with it?"

"Remove the wrapping, take off the strip of paper, and place the pad on your underwear like this."

"What do we do with the other underwear?"

"We wash them."

"Ewww."

"I know. When I was a teenager up until my early twenties, I used to throw my underwear away and buy new ones, if I didn't want to wash them. I thought it was unsanitary to touch the blood. So, we will wash these out and put them in the washer. You can set aside underwear just for your period."

As I was washing out the underwear, I asked Banvoa if this was the first time, she noticed the blood and she said, "No."

I was stunned and felt a little let down. I asked, "When and why didn't you tell me?

"It was Monday and it was just a little stain. I was trying to figure it out myself."

I said, "Okay," and felt a little comforted by her attempt to figure it out herself. It's her body.

After we left the powder room, we sat in the family room, and I explained to Banvoa that she was now a woman and could have babies.

We talked about the period cycle, counting days, keeping her body clean, drinking herbal tea, and paying attention to how her body feels during her cycle and before. After I explained all of that, she slumped down into the chair and said, "Wow. I'm tired." I said, "Yeah. I know. Don't worry, you'll get used to it. You will have your period for a long time. More than 50 years. No, I am just joking. It will just seem like it. We then called the friends and family who participated in her Flowering Party to share the good news. Banvoa was so gleefully proud to announce that she was now a woman.

"Hey, Tiara, it's Banvoa. I'm a woman now."

We were on the phone until after eight that evening. It was a wonderful time of sharing. After I got off the telephone, I shared with Armel that Banvoa started her period and how it happened. He said, "Wow!" He then told me that on Monday morning, Banvoa was complaining about having a headache.

That evening, while lying in bed, I was happy. Happy about my life and, being a mother and. It was an important moment, and I had the support of women, my family, and friends to share it. It was an important transition in Banvoa's life, and I was ready for it—ready to welcome, celebrate, and guide her. I was grateful and thanked the Creator for all our lives.

Every month, during the first year of Banvoa starting her menstrual cycle, I was with her, reminding her to count the days of her cycle, asking how her body felt, and offering her herbs that support the female reproductive system. Herbs such as dong quai, red raspberry, wild yam, and chamomile. It was an intimate time between us. When Banvoa had cramps, we all had cramps. We were so tuned into her sacred time of the month.

After nearly a year, I started thinking more about what I could do as a mother to seal Banvoa's understanding about the sacredness of her body as she continued to physically develop. I thought of how young males offer young ladies promise rings, to promise to be their girlfriends. Well, as a mother, I wanted for Banvoa to make a promise to herself regarding the sacredness of her body and remain abstinent. And so I decided to have a Promise Ring Gathering. Bringing back together Banvoa's sacred circle to expand on what we discussed the previous year.

Well, this is the story of how it all began. Mothers, may you be encouraged to honor your daughters (goddaughters, play daughters) and nieces with a Flowering Party and Promise Ring Gathering? Please remember that sometimes we need stories more than food to keep traveling along our journey. As a woman and mother, I am convinced we need to celebrate the femininity and sacredness of our girl's' bodies for them to know and understand they have nothing to fear or feel embarrassed about because of their menstrual cycle. These treasured memories of being celebrated will strengthen their resolve and anchor them throughout their lives. Their empowerment as they develop into womanhood, at various stages, will help them teach the boys and men how to treat them with love, honor, and respect along their life's journey.

A Word from the Doctor

Eleanor Roosevelt said, "You gain strength, courage, and confidence by every experience in which you really stop to look fear in the face." As a girl starts her menstrual cycle, she has this opportunity. Whether she is nine years old, 16 years old, or any age between, often there is fear of the changes happening to her body as she goes through puberty. Her hips widen, her breasts develop, and hair starts to grow in new places. At some point in, she will look different than all her friends. To make matters worse, her moods go up and down with laughter and tears at the same time. All of which lead up to the start of her menstrual cycle.

Her first period is a scary but natural time. As changes are happening to her body, she has the wonderful chance to talk to the women in her life about their experiences. This sisterhood is a special bond shared by all women. They will have different stories but will have the same ending: a beautiful transition to womanhood. A transition to be embraced not feared.

The first period often starts during times of stress, such as the start of a new school year or during tough exams. The most practical advice, therefore, is to always be prepared. She should carry a panty liner/pad in her purse or book bag. If she does not need it, there is a good chance her friend will. She can always turn to her teacher or school nurse for supplies if necessary – these women will be happy to discretely help her.

Sometimes a girl is afraid she will leave her old self behind – that by growing up, she will no longer be the same person. While the natural processes of puberty are occurring with her body, she is adding to, not losing, her old self. She is a special, wonderful being who has blossomed from a girl to a woman.

After all these changes, she has gained strength, courage, and confidence – all of which she can share with her friends to help them with their fears. The cycle of women bonding into sisterhood continues.

Pediatrician, Dr. Susan Dyar

Note: Dr. Dyar frequently recommends mothers and daughters read together the book, "The Care and Keeping of You," offered by American Girl.

Approximately 70% of women of menstruating age use tampons. A woman may use 11,400 tampons in her life.

BASIC BIOLOGY: THE CYCLE BEGINS

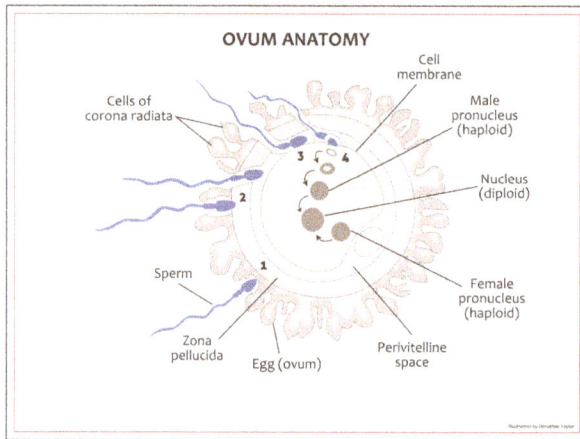

OVUM ANATOMY

"Did you know that when a baby girl is born, she has all the eggs her body will ever use, and many more, as many as 450,000? They are stored in her **ovaries**, each inside its own sac called a **follicle**. As she matures into puberty, her body begins producing various hormones that cause the eggs to mature. This is the beginning of her first cycle; it is a cycle that will repeat throughout her life until the end of menopause.

Let's start with the **hypothalamus**. The hypothalamus is a gland in the brain responsible for regulating the body's thirst, hunger, sleep patterns, libido, and endocrine functions. It releases the chemical messenger **Follicle Stimulating Hormone Releasing Factor (FSH-RF)** to tell the pituitary, another gland in the brain, to do its job. The pituitary then secretes **Follicle Stimulating Hormone (FSH)** and a little **Luteinizing Hormone (LH)** into the bloodstream which cause the follicles to begin to mature.

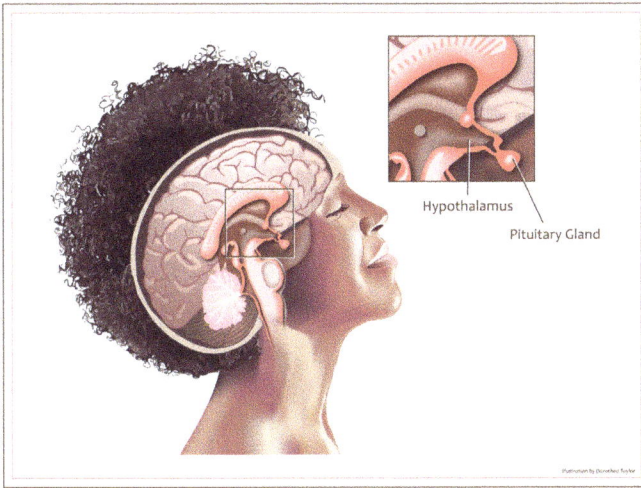

Hypothalamus

Pituitary Gland

The maturing follicles then release another hormone, **estrogen**. As the follicles ripen over a period of about seven days, they secrete more estrogen into the bloodstream. Estrogen causes the lining of the uterus to thicken. It causes the cervical mucous to change. When the estrogen level reaches a certain point, it causes the hypothalamus to release **Luteinizing Hormone Releasing Factor (LH-RF)** causing the pituitary to release a large amount of **Luteinizing Hormone (LH)**. This surge of LH triggers the one most mature follicle to burst open and release an egg. This is called ovulation. [Many birth control pills work by blocking this LH surge, thus inhibiting the release of an egg.]

A woman will spend approximately 3,500 days menstruating.

OVULATION

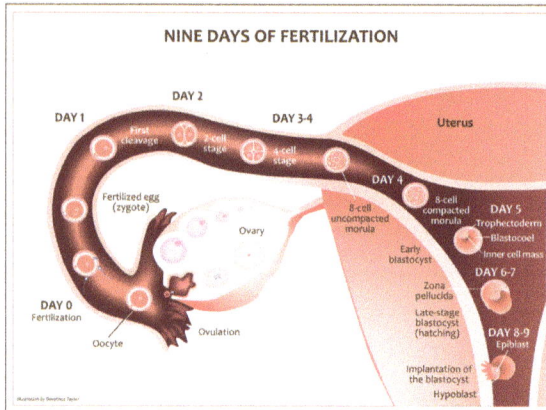

NINE DAYS OF FERTILIZATION

As ovulation approaches, the blood supply to the ovary increases and the ligaments contract, pulling the ovary closer to the Fallopian tube, allowing the egg, once released, to find its way into the tube. Just before ovulation, a woman's cervix secretes an abundance of clear "fertile mucous" which is characteristically stretchy. Fertile mucous helps facilitate the sperm's movement toward the egg. Some women use daily mucous monitoring to determine when they are most likely to become pregnant. The following four points describes the typical progression of the cervical mucus quantity and quality you can expect to see as you move through your menstrual cycle:

1. **After your menstrual period:** The production of cervical mucus is at its lowest immediately following your period, and some women report "dryness" during this time. But, over the next several days, more mucus will become present, and it will like be yellow, cloudy, or white in color, and somewhat sticky to the touch.

2. **As Your Ovulation Date Approaches:** As you enter your fertile window, your cervical mucus will increase in quantity and moistness. The color may be cream-like in appearance.

3. **At the Time of Ovulation:** In the days immediately preceding ovulation, the production of cervical mucus will be at its highest

and the consistency and color of the mucus will be similar to two egg whites. Once you detect the presence of this fertile-quality cervical mucus, you will know you are in your most fertile days.

4. **After Ovulation:** After ovulation, the quantity of cervical mucus begins to decline and become thicker in consistency.

Mid cycle, some women also experience cramping or other sensations. Basal body temperature rises right after ovulation and stays higher by about .4 degrees Fahrenheit until a few days before the next period.

Inside the Fallopian tube, the egg is carried along by tiny, hair-like projections, called "cilia" toward the uterus. Fertilization occurs if sperm are present. [A tubal pregnancy, called ectopic pregnancy, is the rare situation when a fertilized egg implants or gets lodged outside the uterus. It is a dangerous life-threatening situation if the fertilized egg starts developing and growing into an embryo inside the fallopian tube or elsewhere. The tube will rupture causing internal bleeding and surgery is required.

Walt Disney made a movie about menstruation titled, "The Story of Menstruation" in 1946. It is most likely the first film to use the word "vagina."

UTERINE CHANGES

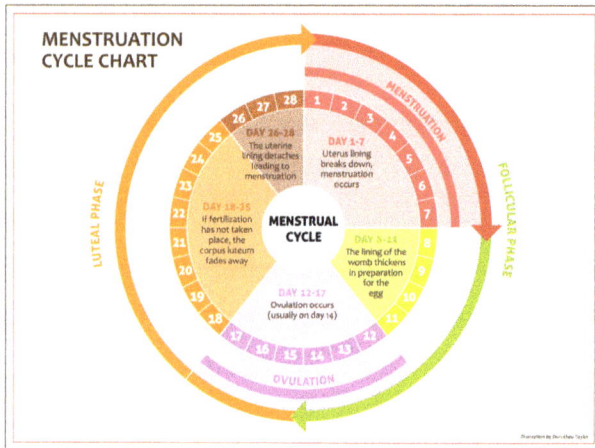

MENSTRUATION CYCLE CHART

Between mid-cycle and menstruation, the follicle from which the egg burst becomes the corpus luteum (yellow body). As it heals, it produces the hormones estrogen and, in larger amounts, progesterone necessary for the maintle turns white and is called the corpus albicans. Estrogen and progesterone are sometimes called "female" hormones, but both men and women have them, just in different concentrations.

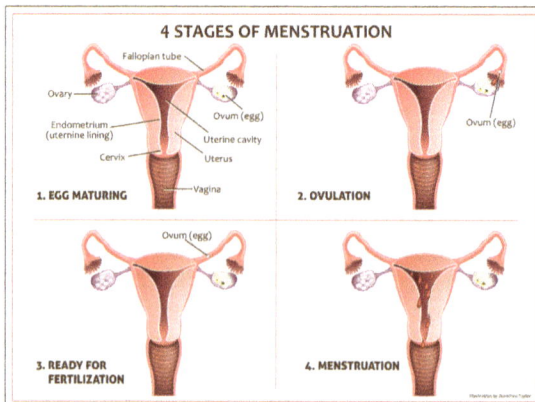

4 STAGES OF MENSTRUATION

*The only mammals to undergo menopause are elephants,
humpback whales, and human females.*

Progesterone causes the surface of the uterine lining, the endometrium, to become covered with mucous, secreted from glands within the lining itself. If fertilization and implantation do not occur, the spiral arteries of the lining close off, stopping blood flow to the surface of the lining. The blood pools into "venous lakes" which, once full, burst and, with the endometrial lining, form the menstrual flow. Most periods last four to eight days, and this length varies over the course of a lifetime. In this illustration, the menstrual cycle is divided into four stages. First, an egg matures inside the ovary (1), which then releases the egg (2), allowing it to travel through the fallopian tube, where its rests awaiting fertilization (3). If the egg is not fertilized, it is flushed out with the menstrual flow (4).

MENSTRUATION

Menstruation is the vaginal bleeding that occurs in adolescent girls and women as a result of hormonal changes. It normally happens in a predictable pattern, once a month.

Menstruation is part of the menstrual cycle, which helps a woman's body prepare for the possibility of pregnancy each month. The body parts involved in the menstrual cycle include the uterus, cervix, ovaries, fallopian tubes, brain, pituitary gland, and the vagina. Certain body chemicals known as hormones rise and fall during the month, causing the menstrual cycle to occur.

A "normal" menstrual period typically occurs every 28 days, from the first day of a period to the first day of the next. However, this can vary from 22 to 36 days. Each period usually lasts from three to seven days, with the average being five. It may take several years from the start of menstruation for periods to settle into a pattern. Irregular periods are common in early adolescence. Even after adolescence, many factors can throw off the timing of menstruation. These include weight changes, starting a new job or school, and relationship problems.

CRAMPS AND OTHER SENSATIONS

Women can experience a variety of sensations before, during or after their menses. Common complaints include backache, inner thigh pains, bloating, nausea, diarrhea, constipation, headaches, breast tenderness, irritability, and other mood changes. Uterine cramping is one of the most common uncomfortable sensations women may have during menstruation. There are two kinds of cramping. Spasmodic cramping is likely caused by prostaglandins, chemicals affecting muscle tension. Some prostaglandins cause relaxation and some cause constriction. A diet high in linoleic and liblenic acids, found in vegetables and fish, increases the prostaglandins for aiding muscle relaxation.

Dysmenorrhea, the medical term for menstrual cramps, the dull or throbbing pain in the lower abdomen many women experience just before and during their menstrual periods. It can be primary or secondary. Primary dysmenorrhea involves no abnormality. Secondary dysmenorrhea involves an underlying physical cause, such as uterine fibroids, pelvic inflammatory disease, or endometriosis. Signs and symptoms of dysmenorrhea, whether primary or secondary, may include the following:

- dull, throbbing pain in the lower abdomen
- radiating pain to the lower back and thighs
- nausea, loose stools, sweating, and dizziness (though these are much less common)

If menstrual cramps become severe enough to keep a girl from going about her day-to-day routine, she should see a doctor. The doctor will perform a medical history and physical examination, including a pelvic exam, where he or she will look for any abnormalities, signs of infection, and potential causes of secondary dysmenorrheal. In addition, the doctor may request a variety of diagnostic tests, such as imaging tests, laparoscopy, and hysteroscopy. Complications can arise from secondary dysmenorrhea. If pelvic inflammatory disease is present, the fallopian tubes may become scarred and possibly cause later infertility or other reproductive problems. Endometriosis can also lead to fertility problems. Congestive cramping causes the body to retain fluids and salt. To counter congestive cramping, avoid wheat and dairy products, alcohol, caffeine, and refined sugar.

NATURAL OPTIONS TO ALLEVIATE CRAMPING:

- Increase exercise. This will improve blood and oxygen circulation throughout the body, including the pelvis.

- Try not using tampons. Many women find tampons increase cramping.
- Avoid red meat, refined sugars, milk, and fatty foods.
- Eat lots of fresh vegetables, whole grains (especially if you experience constipation or indigestion), nuts, seeds and fruit.
- Avoid caffeine. It constricts blood vessels and increases tension.
- Get a massage.
- Drink ginger root tea (especially if you experience fatigue).
- Put cayenne pepper on food. It is a vasodilator and improves circulation.
- Breathe deeply, relax, notice where you hold tension in your body and let it go.
- Ovarian Kung Fu alleviates or even eliminates menstrual cramps and PMS, it also ensures smooth transition through menopause.

The hormones in our bodies are especially sensitive to diet and nutrition. PMS and menstrual cramping are not diseases, but rather, **symptoms of poor nutrition.**

PREMENSTRUAL SYNDROME OR PMS

PMS has been known by women for many, years. Premenstrual syndrome refers to the collection of symptoms or sensations women experience as a result of high hormone levels before, and sometimes during, their periods. One type of PMS is characterized by anxiety, irritability and mood swings. These feelings are usually relieved with the onset of bleeding.

This type relates to the balance between estrogen and progesterone. If estrogen predominates, anxiety occurs. If there is more progesterone, depression may be a complaint.

Sugar craving, fatigue and headaches signify a different type of PMS. In addition to sugar, women may crave chocolate, white bread, white rice, pastries, and noodles. These food cravings may be caused by the increased responsiveness to insulin related to increased hormone levels before menstruation. In this circumstance, women may experience symptoms of low blood sugar; their brains are signaling a need for fuel. A consistent diet including complex carbohydrates will provide a steady flow of energy to the brain and counter the difficulties of blood sugar variations.

The average woman in a modern industrialized society menstruates 450 times in her life. Conversely, prehistoric women menstruated only 50 times—and today, women in agrarian regions menstruate about 150 times in a lifetime.

MENSTRUAL MYTHS

- *Every woman's cycle is or should be 28 days long.*
- *Every woman will or should bleed every month.*
- *Every woman will or should ovulate every cycle.*
- *If a woman bleeds, she is not pregnant.*
- *A woman cannot ovulate or get pregnant while she is menstruating.*

The above statements are myths. Every woman is different.

It's true most women will have cycles around 28 days. But a woman can be healthy and normal and have just three or four cycles a year. Ovulation occurs about 14-16 days *before* women have their period (not 14 days *after* the start of their period). The second half of the cycle, ovulation to menstruation, is fairly consistently the same length, but the first part changes from person to person and from cycle to cycle. In rare cases, a woman may ovulate twice in a month, once from each ovary.

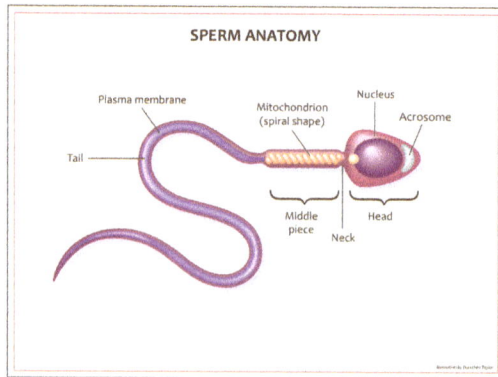

SPERM ANATOMY

Conception/Fertilization of an egg can only occur *after* ovulation. The egg stays alive for about 24 hours once released from the ovary. Sperm can stay alive inside a woman's body for 3-4 days, and possibly as long as 6-7 days. If a couple has intercourse before or after ovulation occurs, they can get pregnant, since the live sperm are already inside the woman's body when ovulation occurs. Thus, a woman can become pregnant from intercourse for about 7-10 days in the middle of her cycle. Fertility Awareness is a birth control method where women monitor their cycles daily to identify ovulation. They predict ovulation to prevent or encourage pregnancy. It requires training and diligent record keeping. In some cases, women can be pregnant and continue to have periods.

MENOPAUSE

Menopause is the last menstrual flow of a woman's life, and the climacteric is period of time preceding and following this event. In general usage, menopause refers to the complete process. For most women, menopause occurs between the ages of forty and sixty and takes place over a period from six months to three years.

The menstrual cycle usually goes through many changes, some slow and some sudden, before stopping altogether. A woman's periods may become erratic, closer together, or farther apart. She may skip a period or two or have spotting at other times in her cycle.

A common experience is loss of substantial amounts of blood with a period and passage of large clots. When a woman nears the cessation of her periods, she may not ovulate for one cycle or several cycles. In this case, the endometrium does not receive the chemical message to stop thickening. It grows until its heavy bulk causes a heavy flow.

Signals of menopause include hot flashes or flushes, changes in sleep patterns, headaches or migraines, high energy, high creativity, and/or mood changes. **As with PMS, some of these symptoms are hormone imbalances caused by poor nutrition.**

Smoking cigarettes can kill a woman's eggs and cause menstrual periods to stop prematurely.

DID YOU KNOW?

- Women lose between 20 and 80 cc's (1-2 ounces) of blood during a normal period.
- One in six fertilized eggs naturally results in miscarriage, some of which are reabsorbed by the body and the woman is not aware she has been pregnant.
- The length of a woman's menstrual cycle (the number of days from the first day of one period to the first day of the next) is determined by the number of days it takes her ovary to release an egg. Once an egg is released, it is about 14 days until menstruation, for nearly all women.

MENSTRUAL HYGIENE PRODUCTS

Once a girl begins menstruating, she needs to choose from the various menstrual hygiene products available. Menstrual hygiene products can be divided into two basic categories: sanitary pads and tampons. Absorbency and comfortable fit are the key features girls need to look for when purchasing menstrual products. Because a girl's menstrual flow may vary from day to day during the cycle, she may want to use several types of products during her period.

Sanitary pads are worn inside the underwear where they collect the menstrual flow. They come in assorted sizes, thicknesses, and styles. Some pads have flaps or "wings" that wrap around and attach to the underside of underwear. Others have deodorant and contain perfume. Some girls find that the perfume irritates their skin.

Tampons are another option for absorbing menstrual flow. Tampons come in various absorbency categories and should be chosen based on the amount of flow experienced. The absorbency of a tampon can be determined by how often it needs to be changed. Girls should use the tampon with the least absorbency necessary to absorb the flow. Tampons should be changed every four to six hours. Tampons also come with a variety of applicators, including plastic and cardboard. Tampons are comfortable to wear and may be an excellent choice for active girls. They should be inserted carefully to avoid any irritation. A rare, but serious, condition called **Toxic Shock Syndrome(TSS)** can be connected to tampon use. The higher the absorbency of tampons used, the higher the risk for TSS. To decrease the risk of TSS, girls should choose the lowest absorbency necessary.

ALTERNATIVES FOR HANDLING MENSTRUAL FLOW

1. Chlorine-free biodegradable 100% cotton tampons recently hit the market in response to environmentally conscious feminists. Studies have shown that organochlorines can be linked to cancer. Women using chlorine-free tampons are not putting chlorine into their bodies, nor are they supporting an industry that produces enormous volumes of industrial waste containing chlorine. If your regular pad or tampon is not chlorine-free, write and urge them to make 100% cotton pads and tampons without chlorine.

2. Natural sponges from the ocean (not cellulose) are used by some women. They are dampened then inserted directly into the vagina. When full, they are removed, washed with water, and reused. Washable reusable cloth pads are also available.

3. The menstrual cap is another reusable alternative. It is similar to the cervical cap but worn near the vaginal opening in the same place as a tampon. When full, it is simply removed, and reinserted. A cervical cap has also been used successfully in this manner.

4. The Keeper—a specially made reusable device for catching monthly flow.

5. Cloth (washable) pads—this is what most women around the word have always used.

To learn more about YOUR OWN cycle, keep a journal or calendar and make note of how you feel, emotionally and physically, thoughts about yourself, your body, your relationships with other cycling women."

The term "period" in reference to menstruation dates from 1822 and means an "interval of time" or a "repeated cycle of events."

REPRODUCTIVE SYSTEM VOCABULARY

As I have said previously, it is especially important to know the names as well as functions of the various parts of the reproductive system. Some children, for whatever reasons, may feel embarrassed by what they do not know. This book offers you a private vocabulary list. You may refer to it in whatever space that offers you comfort to become most familiar with the words and their meanings. A few words have been added because their function supports a process involving the reproductive system. Remember it is important to know YOUR OWN body.

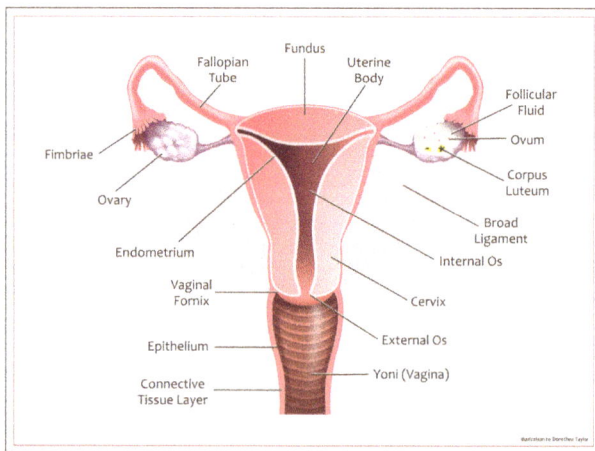

The *female reproductive system* consists of the ovaries, uterus, vagina, and related organs. The two ovaries contain thousands of eggs, and once a month during a female's fertile years, an egg is released into the fallopian tube by one of the two ovaries. If the egg is fertilized, it implants on the wall of the uterus.

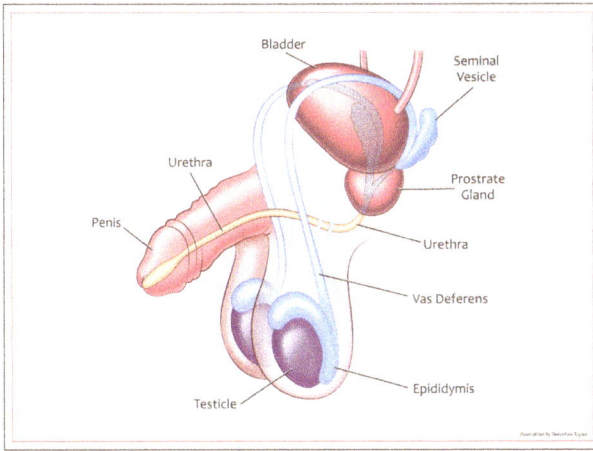

The major parts of the *male reproductive system* include the two testes, suspended in a sac (scrotum) that hangs below the groin and penis. The testes produce sperm and the male sex hormone testosterone. Behind each gland is a tube called the epididymis, which transports the sperm to the urethra for ejaculation through the penis. The prostate and Cowper's gland create the sperm; the sperm is carried in seminal fluid through the urethra from the male to the female reproductive tract during intercourse.

Menstruation may have led to humanity's sense of time as most early lunar (moon) calendars were based on the length of a woman's menstrual cycle.

Abdomen [ab-dōm·ən *or* ab·də,mən] – The abdomen (commonly called the belly) is the body space between the thorax (chest) and pelvis. The diaphragm forms the upper surface of the abdomen. At the level of the pelvic bones, the abdomen ends, and the pelvis begins. The abdomen contains all the digestive organs, including the stomach, small and large intestines, pancreas, liver, and gallbladder. These organs are held together loosely by connecting tissues (mesentery) that allow them to expand and to slide against each other. The abdomen also contains the kidneys and spleen. Many important blood vessels travel through the abdomen, including the aorta, inferior vena cava, and dozens of their smaller branches. In the front, the abdomen is protected by a thin, tough layer of tissue called fascia. In front of the fascia are the abdominal muscles and skin. In the rear of the abdomen are the back muscles.

Abstinence[ab-st-n-ns] — Not having any type of intercourse or sex play with a partner. Abstinence is the only birth control method that is 100% effective in preventing pregnancy as well as sexually transmitted diseases. Being abstinent includes the practice of voluntarily refraining from some or all aspects of sexual activity.

Amenorrhea [ā͵menə-rēə] – The absence of menstrual periods. Primary amenorrhea is the failure to start having a period by the age of 16.

Amniotic Fluid [am-n-o-t-k] [fl-oo-id] – The amniotic sac is filled with the amniotic fluid. This sac is your baby's home, gymnasium, and protection from outside knocks, bumps, and other external pressures. The amniotic sac allows the fetus ample room to swim and move around which helps build muscle tone. To keep the baby cozy, the amniotic sac and fluid maintain a slightly higher temperature than the mother's body, usually 99.7 F. At week 10, there is around 30 ml of fluid present. The amniotic fluid will reach its peak around weeks 34-36 at about one liter. When your water breaks, it is this sac that ruptures and this fluid that leaves the body. Your baby's life is still being supported by the umbilical cord, and you should be meeting your baby soon!

Anus [ā·nəs] — The *anus* is the hole in the middle of your buttocks. The lower opening of the digestive tract. It is associated with the anal sphincter and lies in the cleft between the buttocks, through which fecal (poop) matter is extruded.

Birth Control [bûrth] [kun-trol] — restriction of the number of offspring by means of contraceptive measures; projects, programs, or methods to control reproduction, by either improving or diminishing fertility.

Bladder [bl d r] – A hollow organ in the lower abdomen that stores urine. The kidneys filter waste from the blood and produce urine, which enters the bladder through two tubes, called ureters. Urine leaves the bladder through another tube, the urethra. In women, the urethra is a short tube that opens just in front of the vagina. In men, it is longer, passing through the prostate gland and then the penis. Also known as urinary bladder and vesical.

Some women are heavy, and pass chunks of coagulated blood during their periods. The clots come from uterine contractions and cramping so frequent, the blood doesn't have time to thin out before passing. A few dime-sized or smaller clots a day during a period is normal.

Bloating [blo-t] — is any abnormal general swelling, or increase in diameter of the abdominal area. As a symptom, the patient feels a full and tight abdomen, which may cause abdominal pain, and sometimes accompanied by increased stomach growling or more seriously the total lack of it.

Blood [bluhd] — The "circulating tissue" of the body; the fluid and its suspended formed elements that are circulated through the heart, arteries, capillaries, and veins; blood is the means by which 1) oxygen and nutritive materials are transported to the tissues, and 2) carbon dioxide and various metabolic products are removed for excretion. Blood consists of a pale yellow or gray-yellow fluid, plasma, in which are suspended red blood cells (erythrocytes), white blood cells (leukocytes), and platelets. See also: arterial blood, venous blood.

Body Cavity [bod-e] [kāv'ĭ-tē] — any of the spaces in the human body that contain organs.

Breast [brest] — Either of the pair of milk-secreting mammary glands extending from the front of the chest in pubescent and adult human females and some other mammals.

Broad Ligament [brôd] [lig-a-ment] — The broad ligament of the uterus is the wide fold of peritoneum that connects the sides of the uterus to the walls and floor of the pelvis.

Buttocks [but-ok] — In humans, either of the two fleshy protuberances forming the lower and back part of the hips; in animals the rump.

Cervix [sər·viks] — Located between the vagina and uterus, the cervix serves as a passageway for menstrual blood on the way out, and semen on the way in. (During childbirth, the cervix slowly thins and opens, allowing the baby to move from the uterus and into the vaginal canal.) The cervix opens, closes, and changes in texture throughout a woman's menstrual cycle.

Cervical Mucus [sər·və·kəl] [myü·kəs] — A mucus secreted by glands found in and around the cervix, cervical mucus changes in consistency throughout a woman's reproductive cycle. Cervical mucus may also be referred to as cervical fluid. The job of cervical mucus is to either prevent anything from entering the uterus through the cervix (by becoming sticky and thick), or to nourish and help transport sperm through the cervix (by becoming more abundant, stretchy, and closer to the consistency of raw egg white).

Circumcision [sûr-kəmsĭzh-en] — Is the surgical removal of the foreskin, the tissue covering the head of the penis. It is an ancient practice that has its origin in religious rites. Today, many parents have their sons circumcised for religious or other reasons. Circumcision is usually performed on the first or second day after birth. During a circumcision, the foreskin is freed from the head of the penis (glans), and the excess foreskin is clipped off. If done in the newborn period, the procedure takes about five to 10 minutes. Adult circumcision takes about one hour. The circumcision heals in five to seven days.

Clitoris [klit-or-is, kli-tôr-is] — A small erectile female organ located within the anterior junction of the labia minora that develops from the same embryonic mass of tissue as the penis and is responsive to sexual stimulation.

Conception [kon-sep-shun] – The act of becoming pregnant—fertilization of an ovum by a spermatozoon. The entity formed by the union of the male sperm and female ovum; an embryo or zygote.

Condom [kon-dum] — A flexible sheath, usually made of thin rubber or latex, designed to cover the penis during sexual intercourse for contraceptive purposes or as a means of preventing sexually transmitted diseases. Condoms were originally used as a contraceptive to prevent unwanted pregnancies. A similar device, consisting of a loose-fitting polyurethane sheath closed at one end that is inserted intravaginally before sexual intercourse. Also known as a "rubber."

Connective Tissue Layer [kuh-nek-tiv] [tish-oo] [ley-er] – A material made up of fibers forming a framework and support structure for body tissues and organs.

Constipation[kon-ste-pa-shun] — Abnormally delayed or infrequent passage of dry hardened feces.

When a girl is born, her complete potential egg supply is born with her. In the womb, she creates about seven million egg cells. At birth, she has two million. By puberty, there are only about 400,000 left, of which fewer than 500 are actually released.

Contraception [käntrə-sepSHən] — the deliberate use of artificial methods or other techniques to prevent pregnancy as a consequence of sexual intercourse. The major forms of artificial contraception are barrier methods, of which the most common is the condom; the contraceptive pill, which contains synthetic sex hormones that prevent ovulation in the female; intrauterine devices, such as the coil, which prevent the fertilized ovum from implanting in the uterus; and male or female sterilization.

Corpus Luteum [kawr-puhs loo-tee-uhm] – A yellow mass of cells that forms from a mature ovarian follicle after ovulation and that secretes progesterone. If fertilization of the egg occurs, the corpus luteum persists for the first few months of pregnancy.

Cowper's Fluid [kou-pers] [floo-id] — Pre-ejaculate (also known as pre-ejaculatory fluid, preseminal fluid, or Cowper's fluid, and colloquially as pre-cum) is the clear, colorless, viscous fluid that emits from the urethra of a man's penis when he is sexually aroused. It is similar in composition to semen, but has some significant chemical differences. The fluid is discharged during arousal, masturbation, foreplay or at an early stage during sex, sometime before the man fully reaches orgasm and semen is ejaculated. It is primarily produced by the bulbourethral glands (Cowper's glands), with the glands of Littre (the mucus-secreting urethral glands) also contributing. Pre-ejaculate contains some chemicals associated with semen.

Cowper's Gland (Bulbourethral Glands) [kou-pers] [¦bəl·bō·yuˊrēth·rəl ,gland] — Also called Cowper's glands, these are pea-sized structures located on the sides of the urethra just below the prostate gland. These glands produce a clear, slippery fluid that empties directly into the urethra. This fluid serves to lubricate the urethra and to neutralize any acidity that may be present due to residual drops of urine in the urethra.

Craving [kra-ving] — An intense, urgent, or abnormal desire or longing.

The human female egg is the largest cell in the human body.
It is the only human cell that can be seen with the naked eye.

Diarrhea[die-r-re-a] — abnormally frequent intestinal evacuations with more or less fluid stools (poop, feces). Diarrhea occurs because more fluid passes through the large intestine (colon) than that organ can absorb.

Dysmenorrhea [dismenə-rēə] — Painful menstruation, typically involving abdominal cramps.

Ectopic Pregnancy [ek-top-e-c] [preg-nen-se] — An ectopic pregnancy (EP) is a condition in which a fertilized egg settles and grows in any location other than the inner lining of the uterus. The vast majority of ectopic pregnancies are so-called tubal pregnancies and occur in the Fallopian tube (98%); however, they can occur in other locations, such as the ovary, cervix, and abdominal cavity. An ectopic pregnancy occurs in about one in 50 pregnancies. A molar differs from an ectopic in that it is usually a mass of tissue derived from an egg with incomplete genetic information that grows in the uterus in a grape-like mass that can cause symptoms to those of pregnancy.

Eggs [eg] — Every woman is born with eggs which, when fertilized, develop into a baby. At birth, women have about one million of these eggs stored in their ovaries. By the time you start menstruating, you probably have about 400 000 eggs available for fertilization. Over time, the number of eggs in your ovaries declines, and you may not release an egg every month. Eventually, as you enter menopause, your body will only have a few hundred eggs left and you will probably not ovulate again due to a change in your hormone levels.

Ejaculation [i̯jak·yə-lā·shən] — Is the ejection of semen (usually carrying sperm) from the male reproductory tract, and is usually accompanied by orgasm. It is usually the final stage and natural objective of male sexual stimulation, and an essential component of natural conception.

*A small percentage of women experience endometrial sparing,
when the body recycles the lining of the uterus instead of
shedding it. Consequently, these women's periods are very
brief and light.*

Embryo [em-bre-o] – An organism in the initial stages of development within the womb.

Endocrine System [en-do-krin, -krin, -krin] [sis-tem] — It influences almost every cell, organ, and function of our bodies. The endocrine system is instrumental in regulating mood, growth and development, tissue function, metabolism, and sexual function and reproductive processes. The foundations of the endocrine system are the hormones and glands.

Endometriosis [endō͵mētrē'ōsis] — a condition resulting from the appearance of endometrial tissue outside the uterus and causing pelvic pain.

Endometrium Uterine Lining [en-do-me-tre-em] [yoo-ter-in [lahyning] – The mucous membrane that lines the uterus; thickens under hormonal control and if pregnancy does not occur, is sheds in menstruation; if pregnancy does occur, it sheds with the placenta in at parturition.

Epididymis [ep·ə-did·ə·məs] — The epididymis is a long, coiled tube that rests on the backside of each testicle. It transports and stores sperm cells produced in the testes. It also is the job of the epididymis to bring the sperm to maturity, since the sperm that emerge from the testes are immature and incapable of fertilization. During sexual arousal, contractions force the sperm into the vas deferens.

Epithelium [ep-*uh*-thee-lee-*uh*m] – Tissue that covers a surface, or lines a cavity or the like, and that, in addition, performs any of various secretory, transporting, or regulatory functions.

Estrogen [estrəjən] — A female steroid hormone produced by the ovaries and, in lesser amounts, by the adrenal cortex, placenta, and male testes. Estrogen helps control and guide sexual development, including the physical changes associated with puberty. It also influences the course of ovulation in the monthly menstrual cycle, lactation after pregnancy, aspects of mood, and the aging process. Production of estrogen changes naturally over the female lifespan, reaching adult levels with the onset of puberty (menarche) and decreasing in middle age until the onset of menopause. Estrogen deficiency can lead to lack of menstruation (amenorrhea), persistent difficulties associated with menopause (such as mood swings and vaginal dryness), and osteoporosis in older age. In cases of estrogen deficiency, natural and synthetic estrogen preparations may be prescribed. Estrogen is also a component of many oral contraceptives. An overabundance of estrogen in men causes development of female secondary sexual characteristics (feminization), such as enlargement of breast tissue.

External Orifice Os [ik-stur-nl] [awr-*uh*-fis] or (Ostium) [os-tee*uh*m] – The vaginal opening of the uterus.

Fallopian Tube [fə-lō·pē·ən tüb] — One of the two Fallopian tubes that transport the egg from the ovary to the uterus (the womb). These tubes bear the name of Gabriele Falloppio (also spelled Falloppia), a 16th-century (c. 1523-62) Italian physician and surgeon who was expert in anatomy, physiology, and pharmacology.

Female Reproductive System [fee-meyl] [ree-pr*uh*-duhk-tiv] [sist*uh*m] — is designed to conduct several functions. It produces the female egg cells necessary for reproduction, called the ova or oocytes. The system is designed to transport the ova to the site of fertilization. Conception, the fertilization of an egg by a sperm, normally occurs in the fallopian tubes. The next step for the fertilized egg is to implant into the walls of the uterus, beginning the initial stages of pregnancy. If fertilization and/or implantation does not take place, the system is designed to menstruate (the monthly shedding of the uterine lining). In addition, the female reproductive system produces female sex hormones that maintain the reproductive cycle.

Fertile [fûr-tl] — Capable of reproducing.

Fertilized [fûrtl-iz] — The union of male and female gametes to form a zygote.

Fetus [fe-tus] — An unborn offspring, from the embryo stage (the end of the eighth week after conception, when the major structures have formed) until birth.

Follicle Fluid [fol-i-k*uh*l] [floo-id] – A follicle is a fluid-filled sac that contains an immature egg, or oocyte.

Oligomenorrhea is when a woman has her periods less frequently than normal. Amenorrhea is when she doesn't get her period at all.

Follicle Stimulating Hormone [¦făl·ə·kəl ¦stim·yə,lād·iŋ hȯr,mōn] — A gonadotropic hormone of the anterior pituitary gland that stimulates the growth of follicles in the ovary and induces the formation of sperm in the testis.

Follicle Stimulating Hormone Releasing Factor (FSH-RF) [fol-ik*uh*l] [stim-y*uh*-leyt-ng] [hawr-mohn] [ree-lees-ng] [fak-ter] — a hormone from the hypothalamus that stimulates the synthesis and release of FSH and luteinizing hormone from the anterior pituitary.

Foreskin (Prepuce) [fȯr-skin] ['prēp·əs] — The fold of skin, covering the head (the glans) of the penis. Also called the prepuce.

Fundus [fuhn-d*uh*s] – The upper rounded extremity of the uterus above the openings of the fallopian tubes.

Gametes ['gæmiːt gə-miːt] – Gametes are reproductive cells that unite during sexual reproduction to form a new cell called a zygote. In humans, male gametes are sperm and female gametes are ova (eggs). Sperm are motile and have a long, tail-like projection called a flagellum. Ova, however, are non-motile and relatively large in comparison to the male gamete. Gametes are produced by a type of cell division called meiosis. They are haploid, meaning that they contain only one set of chromosomes. When the haploid male and female gametes unite in a process called fertilization, they form what is called a zygote. The zygote is diploid and contains two sets of chromosomes.

Glans [glanz] – Small rounded body or gland-like mass, such as the head of the penis (glans penis) or clitoris.

Genitalia [jen-i-ta-le-e, -tal-yea] — The sexual organs of reproduction, especially the external organs. Such as the testicles and penis of a male; and the labia, clitoris, and vagina of a female.

Gestation [je-stāSHən] — The process of carrying or being carried in the womb between conception and birth.

Menstruation is the shedding of the uterine lining, or the endometrium. It is the most visible phase of the menstrual cycle.

Gonadotropin-Releasing Hormone Family [go-nad-e-tropin-riles-ing] [hor-mōn] – Are a family of peptides that play a pivotal role in reproduction. The main function of GnRH is to act on the pituitary to stimulate the synthesis and secretion of luteinizing and follicle-stimulating hormones, but GnRH also acts on the brain, retina, sympathetic nervous system, gonads, and placenta in certain species. There seems to be at least three forms GnRH. The second form is expressed in midbrain and seems to be widespread. The third form has been found so far only in fish. GnRH s a C-terminal amidated decapeptide processed from a larger precursor protein. Four of the ten residues are perfectly conserved in all species where GnRH has been sequenced.

Hormones [hor-mo-n] – As the body's chemical messengers, hormones transfer information and instructions from one set of cells to another. Many different hormones move through the bloodstream, but each type of hormone is designed to affect only certain cells.

Human Chorionic Gonadotropin (hCG) [hy-oo-men] [kôr-e-on, kor—] [go-nad-etr-opin, -trop in] – hCG is a hormone produced during pregnancy.

Hypothalamus [hi-po-thal-a-mus] – A region of the brain, between the thalamus and the midbrain, that functions as the main control center for the autonomic nervous system by regulating sleep cycles, body temperature, appetite, etc. And act as an endocrine gland by producing hormones, including the releasing factors that control the hormonal secretions of the pituitary gland.

Infertile [in-fûr-tl] – Absent or diminished fertility. The persistent inability to conceive a child.

Ancient Egyptians (Kemetians) used softened papyrus as rudimentary tampons. Hippocrates notes that the Greeks used lint wrapped around wood. The modern tampon was invented by Dr. Earle Haas in 1929, which was called a "catamenial device" or "monthly device." He trademarked the brand named Tampax.

Internal Orifice[in-tur-nl][awr-*uh*-fis, orInternal (Ostium) [os-teeuhm] – The internal opening of the cervical canal.

Labia Majora [laa-be-e] [me-jôr-e, -jor-e] — The two outer rounded folds of adipose tissue that lie on either side of the vaginal opening and that form the external lateral boundaries of the vulva.

Labia Minora [laa-be-e][me-nôr-e -nor-e] — The inner folds of skin of the external female genitalia.

Labioscrotal — Relating to or being a swelling or ridge on each side of the embryonic rudiment of the penis or clitoris, which develops into one of the scrotal sacs in the male and one of the labia majora in the female.

Luteinizing Hormone (LH) [lüd·ē·ə,nīz·iŋ hôr,mōn] — LH is a hormone secreted by the pituitary gland. It, along with FSH, helps a woman's egg mature and develop. There is a surge of LH right before ovulation that triggers the egg's release from the ovary, and this surge is what at-home ovulation predictor kits look for. In men, LH participates in the production of testosterone, which in turn affects sperm cell growth and development.

Luteinizing Hormone Releasing Factor (LH-RF) [ˈlüd·ē·ə,nīz·iŋ hôr,mōn] — produced by the anterior lobe of the pituitary gland that stimulates ovulation and the development of the corpus luteum in the female and the production of testosterone by the interstitial cells of the testis in the male.

Male Reproductive System [meyl] [ree-pr*uh*-duhk-tiv][sis-t*uh*m] — The entire male reproductive system is dependent on hormones, chemicals that regulate the activity of many distinct types of cells or organs. The primary hormones involved in the male reproductive system are follicle-stimulating hormone, luteinizing hormone, and testosterone. Most of the male reproductive system is located outside of the body. These external structures include the penis, scrotum, and testicles.

Follicle-stimulating hormone is necessary for sperm production (spermatogenesis), and luteinizing hormone stimulates the production of testosterone, also needed to make sperm. Testosterone is responsible for the development of male characteristics, including muscle mass and strength, fat distribution, bone mass, facial hair growth, voice change, and sex drive.

Menarche [men,ärkē] — The time in a girl's life when menstruation first begins. During the menarche period, menstruation may be irregular and unpredictable. Also known as female puberty.

Menorrhagia [menə'rāj(ē)ə] —Abnormally heavy bleeding at menstruation.

Menstruation (Menses)[men-stroo-ashun] [men-sez] — Menstruation is the vaginal bleeding that occurs in adolescent girls and women as a result of hormonal changes. It normally happens in a predictable pattern, once a month. Menstruation is part of the menstrual cycle, which helps a woman's body prepare for the possibility of pregnancy each month. The parts of the body involved in the menstrual cycle include the uterus and cervix, the ovaries, fallopian tubes, the brain and pituitary gland, and the vagina. Certain body chemicals known as hormones rise and fall during the month, causing the menstrual cycle to occur.

Menstrual Cramps [men-stroo-el] [kramp] —Menstrual pain, or menstrual cramps, are caused by the contraction of the uterus. Low abdominal pain that may range from a colicky feeling to a constant dull ache. For these girls, the pain brings aches in the lower back, the abdomen, the pelvic area, and sometimes even in the upper thighs. Fortunately, most menstrual discomfort is normal, but there are times when the pain can be associated with disease or other gynecological problems. The pain may radiate to the lower back and legs. Menstrual cramps are often associated with the beginning of menses, reaching a peak in 24 hours and subsiding after two days.

*Tampon is French for "plug" or "bung," a variant from the
Old French tampon meaning a "piece of cloth to stop a hole."
Before the creation of tampons in the 1920's, Western women
used reusable rags. Some scholars suggest that premodern
women just bled into their clothes, especially since they had
fewer menstrual cycles than modern women.*

Menstrual Cycle [men-stroo-el] [si-kel] — The word menstruation (say men-strew-ay-shun) comes from a Latin word "mens", which means month. The monthly cycle of changes in the ovaries and the lining of the uterus (endometrium), starting with the preparation of an egg for fertilization. When the follicle of the prepared egg in the ovary breaks, it is released for fertilization and ovulation occurs. Unless pregnancy occurs, the cycle ends with the shedding of part of the endometrium, which is menstruation. Although it is the end of the physical cycle, the first day of menstrual bleeding is designated as "day one" of the menstrual cycle in medical parlance.

Mitochondria [mi-te-kon-dre-e] — Mitochondria are self-replicating organelles that play a significant role in generating energy for the cell. They are therefore, called powerhouse of the cell.

Newborn [noo-bawrn] — An infant (from the Latin word *infans*, meaning "unable to speak" or "speechless") is the very young offspring of a human or other mammal. When applied to humans, the term is usually considered synonymous with baby, but the latter is commonly applied to the young of any animal. When a human child learns to walk, the term *toddler* may be used instead.

Oligomenorrhea [ol-i-gō-men-ō-rē-ă] – In frequent or noticeably light menstruation. With oligomenorrhea, menstrual periods occur at intervals of greater than 35 days, with only four to nine periods in a year.

A girl's first menstrual period is called a menarche (from the Greek word men = month + arkhe = beginning). After the menarche, ovulation does not usually occur with menstruation for approximately the first year to 18 months.

Orgasm [ȯr,gaz·əm] — An orgasm is the intense feeling of physical pleasure that humans experience at the climax of sexual stimulation. It is the climax of sexual excitement, experienced as an intensely pleasurable sensation caused by a series of strong involuntary contractions of the muscles of the genital organs. Both men and women can have an orgasm: men need to orgasm to deposit sperm near the cervix, but women do not necessarily need an orgasm to get pregnant.

Ovary [ōv·ə·rē] — One of two female reproductive organs. In women, ovaries are almond-sized organs located in the pelvis, within a fibrous band next to the uterus. Their purpose is to produce and release eggs for fertilization. Ovaries produce sex hormones such as estrogen, progesterone and, in lesser amounts, testosterone. During menopause, the ovaries become less and less active, although they continue to produce some hormones well beyond the end of menses.

Oviduct [oh-vi-duhkt] (Fallopian Tubes) – Transport the egg from an ovary to the uterus (womb).

Ovulation [ăv·yə-lā·shən] — Ovulation refers to the time when the ovary releases an egg for fertilization. It happens once a month and is a distinct stage of your menstrual cycle. Usually, one egg is released from your ovary about two weeks before your period. For most women with a 28-day cycle, ovulation occurs on or around the 14th day. Some women have shorter or longer cycles, ranging anywhere from 21 to 35 days. Ovulation usually occurs sooner if you have a short cycle and later if you have a long cycle. Ovulation is regulated by special hormones released by various parts of your body. Your brain contains hormones that stimulate the growth and development of your eggs. Your ovaries contain female sex hormones like estrogen and progesterone, which help to release eggs during ovulation. It is the interplay between these hormones that triggers ovulation and menstruation. The ovulation cycle is dependent upon signals sent by your body. These signals are sent in the form of changing hormone levels; as your hormone levels increase and decrease, your body responds by triggering separate phases of your menstrual cycle. Ovulation is dependent on signals sent from three main parts of your body:

- the hypothalamus (found in the brain)
- the pituitary gland (found at the base of the brain, near the spine)
- the ovaries (located on either side of your uterus)

Penis [pe·nis] – This is the male organ used in sexual intercourse. Male sex organ, which also provides the channel for urine to leave the body. It has three parts: the root, which attaches to the wall of the abdomen; the body, or shaft; and the glans, which is the cone-shaped part at the end of the penis. The glans, also called the head of the penis, is covered with a loose layer of skin called foreskin. This skin is sometimes removed in a procedure called circumcision. The opening of the urethra, the tube that transports semen and urine, is at the tip of the penis. The penis also contains a number of sensitive nerve endings. The body of the penis is cylindrical in shape and consists of three circular shaped chambers. These chambers are made up of special, sponge-like tissue. This tissue contains thousands of large spaces that fill with blood when the man is sexually aroused. As the penis fills with blood, it becomes rigid and erect, which allows for penetration during sexual intercourse. The skin of the penis is loose and elastic to accommodate changes in penis size during an erection.

Parturition [pärCHoŏ'riSHən] – The action of giving birth to young; childbirth.

Pelvic Cavity ['pel·vik kav·əd·ē] – The pelvic cavity is a body cavity that is bounded by the bones of the. Its oblique roof is the pelvic inlet (the superior opening of the pelvis). Its lower boundary is the pelvic floor. The pelvic cavity primarily contains reproductive organs, the urinary bladder, the pelvic colon, and the rectum.

Pelvis [pel·vəs] – Structure shaped like a funnel in the outlet of the kidney into which urine is discharged before passing into the ureter.

Phallus [fal·əs] – The penis, clitoris, or the sexually undifferentiated embryonic organ out of which either of these develops.

Phytoestrogen [fītō'estrəjən] – an estrogen occurring naturally in legumes, considered beneficial in some diets.

Nicknames for a menstrual period include Aunt Flo, On the Rag, I'm at a Red Light, Surfing the Crimson Tide, checked into the Red Roof Inn, Curse of Dracula, Leak Week, My Dot, and Monthly Oil Change.

Pituitary Gland [pi-too—i-ter-e, -too-] [gland] — A small oval endocrine gland attached to the base of the vertebrate brain and consisting of an anterior and a posterior lobe, the secretions of which control the other endocrine glands and influence growth, metabolism, and maturation.

Placenta [ple-sen-ta] — The placentais a pancake-shaped organ that attaches to the inside of the uterus and is connected to the fetus by the umbilical cord. The placenta produces pregnancy-related hormones, including chorionic gonadotropin (hCG), estrogen, and progesterone. The placenta is responsible for working as a trading post between the mother's and the baby's blood supply. Small blood vessels carrying the fetal blood run through the placenta, which is full of maternal blood. Nutrients and oxygen from the mother's blood are transferred to the fetal blood, while waste products are transferred from the fetal blood to the maternal blood, without the two blood supplies mixing.

Pregnancy [preg·nən·sē] — Process of human gestation that takes place in the female's body as a fetus develops from fertilization to birth (*see* parturition). It begins when a viable sperm from the male and egg from the ovary merge in the fallopian tube (*see* fertilized). The fertilized egg (zygote) grows by cell division as it moves toward the uterus, where it implants in the lining and grows into an embryo and then a fetus. A placenta and umbilical cord develop for nutrient and waste exchange between the circulations of mother and fetus. A protective fluid-filled amniotic sac encloses and cushions the fetus.

Premenstrual Syndrome (PMS) [pre-men-stroo-el] [sin-drom] — has a wide variety of symptoms, including mood swings, tender breasts, food cravings, fatigue, irritability and depression. An estimated three of every four menstruating women experience some form of premenstrual syndrome. These problems tend to peak during your late 20s and early 30s. Symptoms tend to recur in a predictable pattern. Yet the physical and emotional changes you experience with premenstrual syndrome may be particularly intense in some months and only slightly noticeable in others.

Progesterone [projes-te-ron] — A female hormone, the principal hormone that prepares the uterus to receive and sustain fertilized eggs. A steroid hormone, C21H30O2, secreted by the corpus luteum of the ovary and by the placenta, which acts to prepare the uterus for implantation of the fertilized ovum, to maintain pregnancy, and promote development of the mammary glands. Progesterone levels increase in the second half of the menstrual cycle, after ovulation, and usually remain high if the woman gets pregnant. Progesterone helps to maintain the lining of the uterus in order to support a pregnancy.

Prostate Gland [pros-tat] [gland] — The prostate gland is a walnut-sized structure located below the urinary bladder in front of the rectum. The prostate gland contributes additional fluid to the ejaculate. Prostate fluids also help to nourish the sperm. The urethra, which carries the ejaculate to be expelled during orgasm, runs through the center of the prostate gland.

Puberty [pju:bəti] — Puberty is a normal phase of development occurring when a child's body transitions into an adult and readies for the possibility of reproduction. The period or age at which a person is first capable of sexual reproduction of offspring. Physical signs that a girl is entering puberty include growth spurts, breast development, underarm and pubic hair growth, facial acne, body odor, and menstruation. Physical signs that a boy is entering puberty include a deepening of the voice, muscle growth, pubic hair growth, acne, underarm growth, growth spurts, adult body odor, growth of testicles and penis, wet dreams or the ability to ejaculate. It may take two to four years before your tween's body fully transitions through puberty. Girls traditionally enter puberty earlier than boys, and it is common for girls to begin showing signs as early as age nine. For most girls, menstruation may begin around the ages of 11 or 12. Girls who show signs of puberty before the age of eight are known to have precocious puberty, which is a treatable condition that should be evaluated by her health care provider. For boys, the first signs of puberty are likely to occur around the ages of 11 or 12.

*A tampon does not make a woman bleed more than
if she uses a pad.*

Pubic Bone [py-oo-bk] [bon] — One of the three sections of the hipbone; together these two bones form the front of the pelvis.

Rectum [rek·təm] — The rectum is about eight inches long and serves as a warehouse for (feces). It hooks up with the sigmoid colon to the north and with the anal canal to the south. The rectum has little shelves in it called transverse folds. These folds help keep stool in place until you are ready to go to the bathroom. When you are ready, stool enters the lower rectum, moves into the anal canal, and then passes through the anus on its way out.

Reproductive System [rē·prə¦dək·tiv ,sis·təm] — The system of organs and parts which function in reproduction consisting in the male especially of the testes, penis, seminal vesicles, prostate, and urethra and in the female, especially of the ovaries, fallopian tubes, uterus, vagina, and vulva.

Sanitary Pads [san-i-ter-e] [pad] — A disposable pad of absorbent material worn to absorb menstrual flow.

Scrotum [skrōd·əm] — This is the loose pouch-like sac of skin that hangs behind and below the penis. It contains the testicles (also called testes), as well as many nerves and blood vessels. The scrotum acts as a "climate control system" for the testes. For normal sperm development, the testes must be at a temperature slightly cooler than body temperature. Special muscles in the wall of the scrotum allow it to contract and relax, moving the testicles closer to the body for warmth or farther away from the body to cool the temperature.

Secrete [se-kret] — To generate and separate (a substance) from cells or bodily fluids.

Semen [sē·mən] — Which contains sperm (reproductive cells), is expelled (ejaculated) through the end of the penis when the man reaches sexual climax (orgasm). When the penis is erect, the flow of urine is blocked from the urethra, allowing only semen to be ejaculated at orgasm.

Seminal Vesicle [sem·ən·əl ves·i·kəl] — The seminal vesicles are sac-like pouches that attach to the vas deferens near the base of the bladder. The seminal vesicles produce a sugar-rich fluid (fructose) that provides sperm with a source of energy to help them move. The fluid of the seminal vesicles makes up most of the volume of a man's ejaculatory fluid, or ejaculate.

Sperm [spərm] — The term sperm is derived from the Greek word (σπέρμα) *sperma* (meaning "seed") and refers to the male reproductive cells.

Spermatogenesis[spər,mad·ə-jen·ə·səs] — The process of male gamete formation including formation of a spermatocyte from a spermatogonium, meiotic division of the spermatocyte, and transformation of the four resulting spermatids into spermatozoa.

Sexual Intercourse (Copulation [kăp·yə′lā·shən] or Coitus [kō·əd·əs]) — the act carried out for procreation or pleasure in which, typically, the insertion of the male's erect penis into the female's vagina is followed by rhythmic thrusting usually culminating in orgasm.

Tampons [tam-pon] — A plug of absorbent material inserted into a body cavity or wound to check a flow of blood or to absorb secretions, especially one designed for insertion into the vagina during menstruation.

Testicles (Testes) [tes-ti-kel] [tes-tez] — These are oval organs about the size of large olives that lie in the scrotum, secured at either end by a structure called the spermatic cord. Most men have two testes. The testes are responsible for making testosterone, the primary male sex hormone, and for generating sperm. Within the testes are coiled masses of tubes called seminiferous tubules. These tubes are responsible for producing sperm cells.

Testosterone [tes-täs·tə,rōn] — A "male hormone" — a sex hormone produced by the testes that encourages the development of male sexual characteristics, stimulates the activity of the male secondary sex characteristics, and prevents changes in them following castration. Chemically, testosterone is 17-beta-hydroxy-4-androstene-3-one. Testosterone is the most potent of the naturally occurring androgens. The androgens cause the development of male sex characteristics, such as a deep voice and a beard; they also strengthen muscle tone and bone mass. High levels of testosterone appear to promote good health in men, for example, lowering the risks of high blood pressure and heart attack.

It is possible to get pregnant if a woman has vaginal sex during her period because sperm can survive up to a week in the body.

Toxic Shock Syndrome [tok-sik] [shok] [sin-drohm] — Toxic shock syndrome is a severe disease that involves fever, shock, and problems with the function of several body organs. Toxic shock syndrome is caused by a toxin produced by certain types of *Staphylococcus* bacteria. A similar syndrome, called toxic shock-like syndrome (TSLS), can be caused by Streptococcal bacteria. Not all staph or strep infections cause toxic shock syndrome. Although the earliest cases of toxic shock syndrome involved women who were using tampons during their periods (menstruation), today less than half of current cases are associated with such events.

Umbilical Cord[um-bil-i-kel] [kôrd] — Is the lifeline that attaches the placenta to the fetus. The umbilical cord is made up of three blood vessels: two smaller arteries, which carry blood to the placenta and a larger vein, which returns blood to the fetus. It can grow to be 60 cm long, allowing the baby enough cord to safely move around without causing damage to the cord or the placenta. After the baby is born, the cord is cut (something the baby's father may wish to do); the remaining section will heal and form the baby's belly button. During pregnancy, you may find out that the umbilical cord is in a knot or is wrapped around a part of your baby's body. This is common and cannot be prevented, and it usually does not pose any threats to the baby.

Urethra [yə-rē·thrə] — The tube or duct that carries urine from the bladder and out through the penis. Not to be confused with the ureter that carries urine from each kidney to the bladder. In males, it has the additional function of ejaculating semen when the man reaches orgasm. When the penis is erect during sex, the flow of urine is blocked from the urethra, allowing only semen to be ejaculated at orgasm.

Urinary Bladder [yur·ə,ner·ē blad·ər] — The organ that stores urine, which is collected by the kidneys and transferred to the bladder by the ureters. The bladder empties through the urethra, which passes through the prostate gland and then the penis.

Urine [yur·ən] — The liquid-to-semisolid waste matter excreted by the kidneys, in humans being a yellowish, slightly acid, watery fluid.

The same chemicals that cause uterine contractions during menstruation also cause the lower intestine to contract as well, which can lead to diarrhea.

Ureter [yoo-re-ter, yoor-i-ter] – The tube or duct that carries urine from each kidney to the bladder.

Urogenital [yoor-o-jen-i-tl] – Of, relating to, or involving both the urinary and genital structures and functions.

Uterine Lining [yoo-ter-in, -tuh-rahyn] [lahy-ning] – The inner layer of the uterus (womb); the cells that line the womb; endometrium.

Uterus [yoo-ter-uhs] – A hollow, pear-shaped organ located in a woman's lower abdomen, between the bladder and the rectum. The narrow lower portion of the uterus is the cervix (the neck of the uterus). The broader upper part is the corpus, made up of three layers of tissue. In women of childbearing age, the inner layer (endometrium) of the uterus goes through a series of monthly changes known as the menstrual cycle. Each month, endometrial tissue grows and thickens in preparation to receive a fertilized egg. Menstruation occurs when this tissue is not used, disintegrates, and passes out through the vagina. The middle layer (myometrium) of the uterus is muscular tissue that expands during pregnancy to hold the growing fetus and contracts during labor to deliver the child. The outer layer (parametrium) also expands during pregnancy and contracts thereafter.

Vagina [və-jī-nə] – The vagina is a muscular canal extending from the cervix to the outside of the body. The muscular canal that extends from the cervix to the outside of the body. It is usually six to seven inches in length, and its walls are lined with mucous membrane. It includes two vault like structures: the anterior (front) vaginal fornix and the posterior (rear) vaginal fornix. The cervix protrudes slightly into the vagina, and through a tiny hole in the cervix (the os), sperm make their way toward the internal reproductive organs. The vagina also includes numerous tiny glands that make vaginal secretions. The word "vagina" is a Latin word meaning "a sheath or scabbard," a scabbard into which one might slide and sheath a sword. The "sword" in the case of the anatomic vagina was the penis. Love and war, it would seem, have been connected in the minds of people for millennia.

The United States has one of the highest teen pregnancy rates in the western industrialized world.

Vaginal Fornix [vaj-*uh*-nl] [fawr-niks] – A recess in the upper part of the vagina caused by the protusion of the uterine cervix into the vagina.

Vas Deferens ['vas def·ə·rənz] — The vas deferens is a long, muscular tube that travels from the epididymis into the pelvic cavity, to just behind the bladder. The vas deferens transports mature sperm to the urethra, the tube that carries urine or sperm to outside of the body, in preparation for ejaculation.

Vulva [vŭl-və] — The external genital organs of the female, including the labia majora, labia minora, clitoris, and vestibule of the vagina.

Womb [woom] – A hollow muscular organ in the pelvic cavity of females; contains the developing fetus.

X Chromosome [kro-me-som] – A sex chromosome of humans and most mammals that determines femaleness when paired with another X chromosome and that occurs singly in males.

Y Chromosome [kro-me-som] — A Y-chromosome is the sex chromosome found only in males. The two types of sex chromosomes, X and Y, determine the sex of an embryo. Women have two X chromosomes and men have an X and a Y chromosome. Because of this, the sex of the child is determined by the chromosome passed by the male.

Yolk Sac [yok] [sak, sôk] – A structure that develops in the inner cell mass of the embryo and expands into a vesicle with a thick part that becomes the primitive gut and a thin part that grows into the cavity of the chorion. The cells of the extra embryonic mesoderm differentiate to develop endothelium, primitive blood plasma, and hemoglobin. The yolk sac usually disappears during the seventh week of pregnancy.

Yoni [yo-ne] — A term borrowed from India's ancient language, Sanskrit or Devanagari (Skt., divine language). It can be translated by several English concepts (origin, source, womb, female genitals) and is, considered by many, the most respectful word available for naming what in correct language we call vulva (Lat., female genitals, womb) yet which is often (wrongfully) called vagina (Lat., sheath); unless slang is used.

The term yoni heralds from a culture and religion in which women have long been regarded and honored as the embodiment of divine female energy - the goddess known as *Shakti* - and where the female genitals were/are seen as a sacred symbol of the Great Goddess. Because Tantric, and others worship the Divine in the form of a Goddess, the term Yoni has also acquired other, more cosmic meanings, becoming a symbol of the *Universal Womb*, the *Matrix of Generation* and *Source of All*. In short, the universe really is a yoniverse.

Zygote [zi-got] – Is a fertilized egg cell that results from the union of a female gamete (egg, or ovum) with a male gamete (sperm). In the embryonic development of humans and other animals, the zygote stage is brief and is followed by cleavage, when the single cell becomes subdivided into smaller cells. The zygote represents the first stage in the development of a genetically unique organism. The zygote is endowed with genes from two parents, and thus it is diploid (carrying two sets of chromosomes).

NUTRITION FOR A HEALTHY REPRODUCTIVE SYSTEM

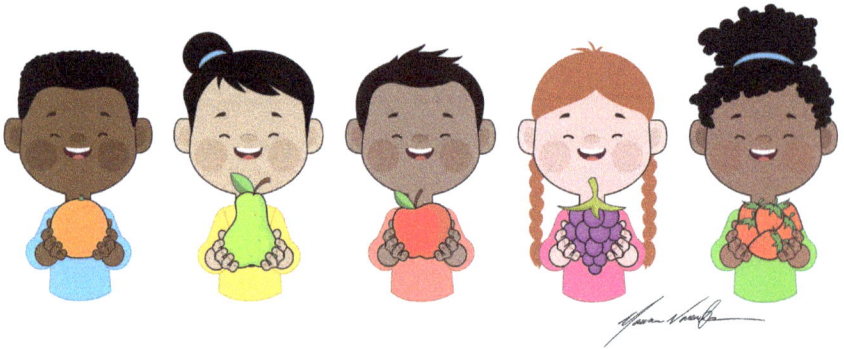

Vitamins, minerals, electrolytes, amino acids, herbs, and water are a prerequisite to a healthy female and male reproductive system. Your body requires a total of 13 essential vitamins to perform several essential functions. If you are not getting proper amounts of these 13 vitamins, you can suffer from deficiency. There is no question that our food choices have undergone dramatic changes in the last 100 years. Eat "naturally from the earth" get plenty of fresh vegetables, fruits, whole grains, legumes, nuts, brown rice, and seeds. Legumes are plants that bare their fruits in pods. For example, black beans, black eye peas, chickpeas (garbanzo beans), kidney beans, fava beans, lima beans, navy beans, mung beans and pinto beans. Do your best to avoid junk food, processed foods, and foods high in saturated fat. Saturated fats are simply fat molecules that have no double bonds between carbon molecules because they are saturated with hydrogen molecules. Saturated fats are typically solid at room temperature.

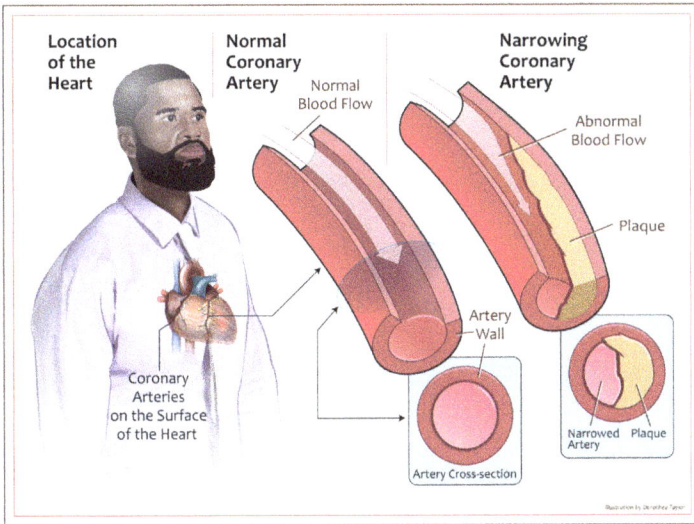

Eating foods that contain saturated fats raises the level of cholesterol in your blood. Elevated levels of LDL (lipoproteins) cholesterol in your blood increase your risk of heart disease and stroke. Lipoproteins are made of fat (lipid) on the inside and proteins on the outside. LDL cholesterol sometimes is called "bad" cholesterol. Processed meats such as sausage, cold cuts, pepperoni, bologna, and hot dogs contain LDL cholesterol, claims the American Heart Association. Other processed foods that contain LDL include breakfast cereals, breads, crackers, energy bars, deep-fried fast foods, many restaurant foods, boxed foods, canned foods, and prepackaged foods. A high LDL level leads to a buildup of cholesterol in your arteries. (Arteries are blood vessels that carry blood from your heart to your body.) For some, it may sound as if I am asking you not to eat. Remember, this section is discussing nutrition, which is vital to healthy functioning of the reproductive system. Because more than not children do their best to avoid certain fruits and vegetables, unaware of the important nutritional facts for eating to live well, health, and strong. Please refer to **United States of Department of Agriculture (USDA) Food and Nutrition Center** at website: http://fnic.nal.usda.gov for more detailed information.

The term "menstruation" is equivalent (equal) to the Old English monad blot or "month blood." In Latin, menses means "month."

WATER

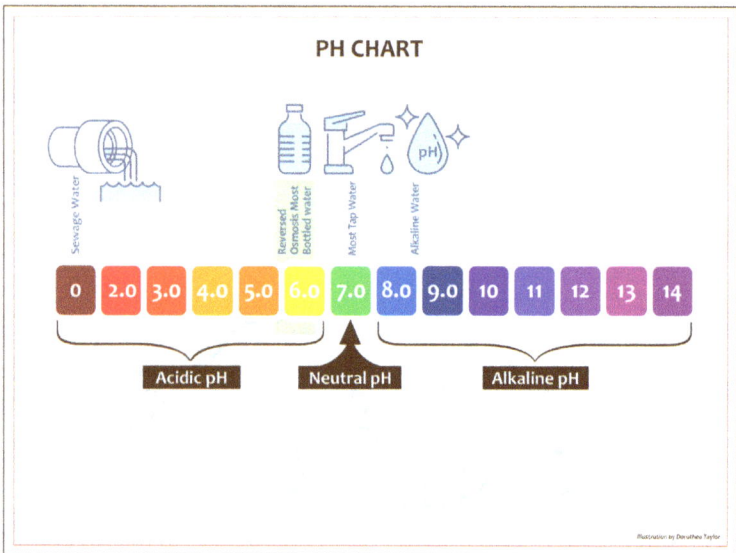

PH CHART

Sewage Water					Reversed Osmosis Most Bottled water		Most Tap Water	Alkaline Water					
0	2.0	3.0	4.0	5.0	6.0	7.0	8.0	9.0	10	11	12	13	14

Acidic pH   Neutral pH   Alkaline pH

Illustration by Dorothea Taylor

According to Dr. David Dyer, author of CELLFOOD Vital Cellular Nutrition for the New Millennium, scientists estimate that humans can live no more than 10 days without water, such is the importance of this element. All chemical reactions in the body take place in water. Every cell in the body is bathed water, which contains materials to keep them vibrant. Water is the transporter of nutrients and oxygen for proper function of the body's tissues; it helps remove waste from the bod, acts as a natural air conditioner through perspiration, is essential for digestion and absorption of vitamins and minerals. Water keeps our skin moist and supple and is a natural lubricant for our joints and internal organs. Drink plenty of water to flush out any toxins in the body and for maintaining hydration (providing an adequate amount of liquid to bodily tissues.) A great formula to use to determine how many daily ounces of water your body needs for hydration is to divide your body weight by two (drink more than your daily allowance to release weight). The body keeps a reserve store of fuel, such as stores of fat, which can be tapped in emergencies, but we have no built-in water tank to tap into when running dry—even though our bodies are 70-80% water! For instance, the brain is 75% water, heart 75%, lungs 86%, muscles 75%, blood 83%, liver 86% and kidneys 83%.

Clean water is essential to our well-being. The growing pollution in our modern-day world is having an increasingly detrimental effect on our drinking water. Hazardous chemicals like mercury, lead, arsenic, cyanide, aluminum, and phosphorus are getting into the water system daily. Other dangerous and toxic chemicals, including chlorine and fluoride, are added to reduce harmful microorganisms and prevent tooth problems. All this adds to the load of toxins that our bodies have to eliminate. For excellent quality drinking water, we need to purify or filter typically available tap water before drinking it. There are many water purification systems to choose from, as well as many types of bottled water using various purification processes. The normal functioning of all the body systems, organs, and glands, including those involved with the menstrual cycle, are affected by the quality of water we drink. When drinking water, please consider the pH (potential for hydrogen or hydrogen power) balance of the water to determine level of acidity or alkalinity. Alkaline means having the properties of an alkali (an ionic salt), or containing alkali; having a pH greater than seven; likewise, acidic means having the properties of an acid, or containing acid; having a pH below seven. Many people believe water with an alkaline level higher than seven offers more health benefits. In your choice for alkalinity, please consider that the human blood pH is 7.4 and that your life is in your blood.

The term "ovary" is from the Latin ovum or "egg." In classical Latin, ovaries meant "egg keeper."

VITAMINS

"Vitamins are organic compounds which are needed in small quantities to sustain life. We get vitamins from food, because the human body either does not produce enough of them or none at all. Vitamins are essential to normal metabolism; insufficient amounts from what we eat may cause deficiency diseases. An organic compound contains carbon. When an organism (living thing) cannot produce enough of an organic chemical compound that it needs in tiny amounts, and has to get it from food, it is called a vitamin. For instance, the body can produce vitamins D and K.

Put simply, a vitamin is both:
1. An organic compound (contains carbon).
2. An essential nutrient the body cannot produce enough of on its own, so it must get it (tiny amounts) from food.

There are *fat-soluble* and *water-soluble* vitamins:

Fat-soluble vitamins are stored in the fat tissues of our bodies, as well as the liver. Fat-soluble vitamins are easier to store than water-soluble and can stay in the body as reserves for days, some for months. Vitamins A, D, E and K are fat-soluble. Fat-soluble vitamins are absorbed through the intestinal tract with the help of fats (lipids).

Water-soluble vitamins do not get stored in the body for long—they soon get expelled through urine. Water-soluble vitamins need to be replaced more often than fat-soluble ones. Vitamins C and all the B vitamins are water-soluble.

There are currently 13 recognized vitamins essential to the body and its functions.

Menstruation huts were common features in premodern cultures. They were a place where women were separated from the community during their menses for various reasons ranging from fear to respect.

Knowing precisely which vitamins positively affect the female and male reproductive system is crucial to maintaining health and well-being. For example, pumpkin seeds are a great food for male fertility, as they contain prominent levels of zinc and essential fatty acids vital to healthy functioning of the male reproductive system.

Vitamin A (Retinol)

Vitamin A can help support a woman's fertility in many ways, most noticeably is it promotes better cervical fluid. Not only can it help your body to produce more fluid, the fluid itself is more nourishing for the sperm and helps them to live longer, allowing for more time to meet the egg. Vitamin A also assists the follicles in maturing properly. Both in the maturation of an egg and in assisting the follicle in producing the hormones needed to aid the fertilized egg into the uterus. Vitamin A is used for heavy menstrual periods, premenstrual syndrome (PMS), vaginal infections, yeast infections, "lumpy breasts" (fibrocystic breast disease), and to prevent breast cancer.

Vitamin A Food Source: Butternut squash, kale, turnip greens, spinach, green, swiss chard, romaine lettuce, dandelion greens, beet greens, pak choi, pumpkin, cantaloupe, papaya, mango, passion fruit, watermelon, guava, tomatoes, grapefruit, leeks, brussel sprouts, Chinese broccoli, pumpkin, dried apricot, sweet red, yellow, and green peppers, sweet potatoes, Chinese cabbage, bok choy, pecans, chestnuts, and pistachios.

Vitamin B1 (Thiamin)

Vitamin B1 helps convert carbohydrates (Carbohydrates are found in almost all living things and play a critical role in the proper functioning of the immune system, fertilization, pathogenesis, blood clotting, and human development.)into energy and is essential for the functioning of the heart, muscles, and nervous system.

Vitamin B1 Food Source: Fortified breads, pasta, wheat germ, macadamia nuts, sunflower seeds, pumpkin seeds, acorn squash, boysenberries, dates, grapes, grapefruit, guava, mango, orange pineapple, pomegranate, watermelon, loganberries, avocado, green peas, asparagus, navy beans, black beans, soy beans (edamame), brazil nuts, black beans, black-eyed peas, white beans, buckwheat, cashews, chestnuts, flax seed, hazelnuts, peanuts, pecans, quinoa, brown rice, pistachios, rye, spelt, lima beans, okra, French beans, potatoes, and spirulina.

Vitamin B2 (Riboflavin)

Vitamin B2 is needed for normal cell function, growth, and energy production.

Vitamin B2 Food Source: Almonds, avocado, banana, grapes, lychee, mango, mulberries, passion fruit, pomegranate, prickly pear, artichoke, asparagus, bok choy, brussel sprouts, lima beans, mushrooms, pumpkin, spirulina, sweet potato, winter squash, quinoa, rye, buckwheat, oats sesame seeds, beet greens, swiss chard, chestnuts, wheat (durum, hard red, hard white), pinto beans, navy beans, garbanzo beans, fava beans, asparagus, brown mushrooms (crimini), spinach, and soy beans (edamame).

Vitamin B3 (Niacin/Nicotinic Acid)

Vitamin B3 is essential for converting food to energy, assists in the functioning of the digestive system, skin, and nerves.

Vitamin B3 Food Source: Spirulina, seaweed, chia seeds, peanut butter, paprika, green peas, sunflower seeds, avocado, broccoli, asparagus, kidney beans, bell peppers, tahini, fortified cereal, shitake and portabella mushrooms, boysenberries, loganberries, lychee, mango, peach, passion fruit, artichoke, dates, guava, butternut squash, mushrooms, okra, parsnip, peas, potatoes, spaghetti squash, pumpkin, spirulina, barley, buckwheat, rye, sunflower seeds, wheat (durum, hard red, hard white), navy beans, pinto beans, mung beans, legumes (Legumes are plants that bare their fruits in pods. Well-known legumes alfalfa, clover, peas, beans, lentils, lupins, mesquite, carob, kidney beans, pinto beans, black eye peas, garbanzo beans, mung beans, soybeans, peanuts, tamarind, and the woody climbing vine wisteria.)

The word taboo comes from the Polyneisain tapua, meaning both "sacred" and "menstruation."

Vitamin B5 (Pantothenic Acid)

Vitamin B5 is essential for growth and metabolism of food and the formulation of hormones as well as (good) cholesterol.

Vitamin B5 Food Source: Avocado, black currants, dates, gooseberries, grapefruit, guava, pomegranate, raspberries, starfruit watermelon, broccoli, brussel sprouts, butternut squash, French beans, mushrooms, okra, pumpkin, spirulina, spaghetti squash, winter squash, whole grain cereals, legumes, white and sweet potatoes, buckwheat, black-eyed peas, soy beans (edamame), lima beans, mung beans, split peas, chestnuts, oats, rye, sunflower seeds, and wheat (durum, hard red, hard white).

Vitamin B6 (Pyridoxine, Pyridoxal, Pyridoxine, Pyridoxamine)

Vitamin B6 is important for protein metabolism, formation of red blood cells and fat usage by your body. Vitamin B6 offers additional support in terms of increased fertility because it balances out the hormone levels. Vitamin B6 focuses mainly on correcting low progesterone levels of women affected by luteal phase defect, in which their luteal phases are not long enough to sustain a successful pregnancy. A normal progesterone level is essential to keep up the pregnancy otherwise it could lead to a miscarriage.

Vitamin B6 Food Source: Banana, bok choy, brussel sprouts, butternut squash, gooseberries, grapes, guava, lychee, mango, passion fruit, pineapple, pomegranate, french beans, green pepper, watermelon, sweet potatoes, kale, lima beans, peas, spirulina, dried prunes, raisins, banana, spaghetti squash, winter squash, chestnuts, hazelnuts, pistachios, pumpkin seeds, sunflower seeds, walnuts, rye, okra, legumes, spinach, avocado, peanut butter, and wheat (durum, hard red, hard white).

Some scientists have suggested harvesting stem cells from menstrual blood.

Vitamin B7 (Biotin/Vitamin H)

Vitamin B7 is essential for growth and metabolism. It is known that the thyroid and adrenal glands, nervous and reproductive systems, and our skin depend on an sufficient supply of this vitamin, Biotin plays a crucial role in metabolizing fats, proteins, and carbohydrates, and several other enzymes involved in the body's metabolic process. It also synthesizes fatty acids, amino acids, keeps blood glucose levels in check, supplements calcium deposits in your nails and keeps them strong, brittle-free.

Vitamin B7 Food Source: Green peas, broccoli, cabbage, cauliflower, sweet potatoes, green and leafy vegetables like spinach, bananas, avocados, strawberries, raspberries, watermelon, grapefruit, oats, soybeans, wheat germ, mushrooms, lentils, split peas, bran, and unpolished brown rice, almonds, pecan, peanuts and walnuts, and brewer's yeast.

Vitamin B9 (Folate/Folic Acid)

Folic acid is an essential vitamin both during pre-conception and pregnancy, as it can prevent spina-bifida in your baby, and other birth defects associated with the brain and spine development in the baby. It used in our bodies to make new cells and helps control blood levels. Also, it is used for protein metabolism, produce DNA, and grow tissues. **In addition, this vitamin promotes sustainable fertility in women and prepares their bodies for pregnancy.** Supplementation with this vitamin is greatly beneficial, since only 50% of the folic acid found in the ingested food can be properly absorbed by the human body.

Vitamin B9 Food Source: Spinach, avocado, blackberries, boysenberries, guava, artichoke, bok choy, buckwheat, chestnuts, rye, quinoa, hazelnuts, peanuts, broccoli, beets, asparagus, beans, legumes, citrus fruits, whole grains, dark green leafy vegetables, mango, loganberries, orange, papaya, pineapple, spirulina, pomegranate, passion fruit, raspberries, soy beans (edamame) strawberries, lima beans, parsnip, romaine lettuce, turnip greens, wheat (durum, hard red, hard white), and sweet potatoes.

Scholars suggest that as matriarchy gave way to patriarchy, menstrual blood taboos were used by men to control women and, consequently, menstrual blood was interpreted away from something powerful to a "disgusting" waste product that had no role in the reproductive process.

Vitamin B12 (Cobalamin)

Vitamin 12 is essential for development of red blood cells, maintenance of nervous system, and metabolism. Deficiency can cause anemia and neurological disorders. **A key vitamin for improved fertility.** Vitamin B12 enhances the occurrence of ovulation, particularly helpful to women not ovulating, making it harder to try to conceive. Vitamin B12 also improves the inner lining of the uterus, creating a favorable environment for the implantation of the fertilized eggs. For men, increases sperm motility and sperm count and helps to increase and boost natural *testosterone* production. It also may help to boost the endometrium lining in egg fertilization, decreasing the chances of miscarriage. Some studies have found that a deficiency of B12 may increase the chances of irregular ovulation, and in severe cases stop ovulation altogether.

Vitamin B12 Food Source: Spirulina, chlorella, blue-green algae, brewer's yeast, fortified soymilk, fortified cereals, and B12 supplements.

Vitamin C (Ascorbic Acid)

This excellent antioxidant also aids in both male and female fertility, given the key part it plays in conception. For men, it helps to keep sperm from clumping together, counteracts the damaging effects of free radicals on the quality of the sperm, and increasing their motility. Also, vitamin helps men maintain healthy testosterone. For women, vitamin C sustains an appropriate female endocrine equilibrium and increases fertility in particular in the case of women having low progesterone levels. It also reinforces the right balance between estrogen and progesterone levels. It will assist with headaches and migraines associated with menopause; and help regulate heavy periods, when combined with bioflavonoids. Vitamin C helps to prevent anemia. During your period, you lose iron as a result of menstrual blood loss. If your period is especially heavy or you have a shorter cycle, you may be at risk for developing iron-deficient anemia, characterized by fatigue and weakness. However, vitamin C allows your body to absorb iron more efficiently, potentially warding off anemia. Clinical trials on women have proven that the chances of getting pregnant doubled following the vitamin C treatment.

Vitamin C Food Source: Oranges, black currants, grapefruit, guava, kiwi, lychee, mango, mulberries, orange, papaya, passion fruit, pineapple, bok choy, brussel sprouts, butternut squash, chestnuts, lemons, limes, clementine, grapefruit, turnip greens, swiss chard, spinach, gold kiwi, broccoli, cranberries, red, yellow, and green peppers, green peas, strawberries, raspberries, blackberries, blueberries, cantaloupe, sweet and white potatoes, and tomatoes.

Vitamin D (calciferol)

Vitamin D is essential to both male and female fertility. It stimulates the levels of estrogen and progesterone, regulates menstruation and improves the viability of sperm, therefore enhancing a successful outcome. Vitamin D helps your body absorb and regulate calcium and phosphorus in the blood; a mineral which may have a protective role against PMS. In addition, vitamin D may help to regulate hormones and help your neurotransmitters, which affect your mood, to function regularly. A study discussed in the July 2010 issue of "The Journal of Steroid Biochemistry and Molecular Biology" examined vitamin D intake among college-aged women and found that women with a high intake of vitamin D from food sources were less likely to have PMS. In addition, Vitamin D is an essential vitamin during pregnancy with studies showing its use vastly decreasing the risk of preterm labor as well as the risk of other pregnancy complications. Vitamin D is needed to help the body create sex hormones, affects ovulation and hormonal balance.

Vitamin D Food Source: Exposure to sunshine, supplements, and mushrooms (crimini, portabella, shitake, oyster).

Because women weigh more than they did in the past, they tend to start their periods at younger ages and stop at older ages (fat cells produce more estrogen). Scholars suggest that hormones in modern food have led to earlier menstruation.

Vitamin E (tocopherol; antioxidant)

Vitamin E is the vitamin of choice for the overall male and female reproductive system. For women, the fertility-friendly vitamin E improves the quality of cervical mucus, thus enhancing the chances of implantation of the fertilized eggs, and, it prolongs the sperm's life within the female a couple more days, to increase the chances for egg fertilization. Vitamin E helps with lumpy and tender breasts and assists with headaches and migraines associated with menopause. If you suffer from cramps, vitamin E may provide you with some relief. According to "MedlinePlus," vitamin E appears to decrease the duration and severity of cramps and may even reduce menstrual blood loss. If you also struggle with menstrual migraines, vitamin E may have additional benefits. A study published in the January 2009 issue of "Medical Science Monitor" found that vitamin E relieved nausea, light sensitivity and sound sensitivity associated with menstrual migraines. Vitamin E helps to improve the overall health of sperm. Sperm can be damaged by harmful molecules (free radicals). Vitamin E is an antioxidant which helps to reduce the number of free radicals. For men, a daily intake of vitamin E is recommended in order to enhance sperm motility.

Vitamin E Food Source: Spinach, asparagus, avocado, orange, mango, papaya, guava, kiwi, nectarine, peach, pomegranate, raspberries, mulberries, tofu, pistachios, turnip greens, collards, kale, cranberries, blueberries, boysenberries, blackberries, black currants, broccoli, butternut squash, potatoes, parsnip, swiss chard, spirulina, green leafy vegetables, almonds, hazelnuts, pine nuts, walnuts, pecans, sunflower seeds, soybeans (edamame) pinto beans, cauliflower, parsley, and banana.

Vitamin K (menaquinone)

Vitamin K is essential for blood clotting and deficiency can cause excessive bleeding. Deficiencies are common in infants or in individuals who take antibiotics or anticoagulants.

Vitamin K Food Source: Collards, cress, spinach, turnip greens, mustard greens, beet greens, swiss chard, scallions, cauliflower, cress, radicchio, brussel sprouts, lettuce, broccoli, cabbage, prunes, pear, plum, raspberries, tomatoes, pomegranate, mulberries, grapes, kiwi, loganberries, avocado, blackberries, blueberries, cranberries, boysenberries, prunes, alfalfa sprouted, artichoke, asparagus, cucumber, kale, leeks, okra, peas, cauliflower, celery, cashews, chestnuts, hazelnuts, pine nuts, pistachio, rye, soy beans (edamame), kidney beans, and split peas."

In many cultures, a fetus was thought to be formed in the womb by clotting menstrual blood.

The 21 Essential Minerals Your Mind and Body Needs

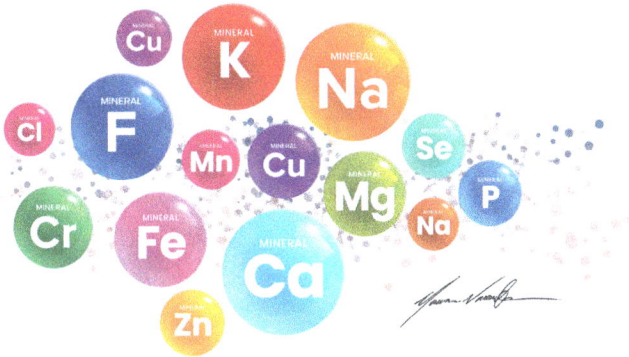

According to Guhu, Ionic Minerals Essential For Your Body And Mind, minerals are necessary for chemical reactions and for building some important molecules in the body. For example, iron is a necessary component of red blood cells, and calcium is essential to maintain the skeleton. Minerals are combined into two groups: Trace Minerals and Major (Macro) Minerals. Trace minerals are minerals your body needs only in tiny amounts each day. They are important for many biological processes for your health. Iron, zinc, copper, selenium, iodine, fluorine, and chromium are Trace Minerals, and the Major (Macro) Minerals, the most important, are minerals your body requires in your diet in abundance for your health. For instance, sodium, potassium, calcium, phosphorus, magnesium, manganese, sulfur, cobalt, and chlorine are Major (Macro) Minerals.

MINERALS SERVE THREE ROLES:

1. They provide structure in forming bones and teeth,
2. They help maintain normal heart rhythm, muscle contractility, neural conductivity, and acid-base balance,
3. They help regulate cellular metabolism by becoming part of enzymes and hormones that modulate cellular activity.

Minerals are necessary for chemical reactions and building important molecules in the body. For example, iron is a necessary component of red blood cells, and calcium is essential to maintain the skeleton. These are 21 minerals maintain health, and typically, only tiny amounts are needed for good health. Plants absorb minerals from the soil, and animals get their minerals from the plants or other animals they eat. Most of the minerals in the human diet come directly from plants, such as fruits and vegetables, or indirectly from animal sources. Minerals may also be present in your drinking water, but this depends on where you live, and the water you drink (bottled, tap). Minerals from plant sources may also vary from place to place, because the mineral content of the soil varies according to the location the plant was grown.

BORON (B) – Trace Mineral

Builds strong healthy bones and muscles as well as helps prevent bone loss. It aids in improving the thinking function.

Boron Food Source: Leafy green vegetables, legumes, red apples, carrots, grapes, nuts, pears, whole grains, raisins, prunes, peanuts, honey, broccoli, bananas, chickpeas, onions, oranges, walnuts, almonds, avocados, pears, green beans, hazelnuts, dandelion, parsley, pig weed, cabbage, and garlic.

CALCIUM (Ca) – Major Mineral

Insufficient calcium in the body can affect the bones which can lead to osteoporosis, high blood pressure and colon cancer. Another effect involves sensations of numbness and tingling around the mouth and fingertips and painful aches and spasms of the muscles. Having enough calcium can ease the symptoms of premenstrual syndrome (PMS). An adequate supply of calcium helps muscles, including the heart, to contract and relaxing. Calcium also appears to help regulate pressure in arteries to the nervous system.

The family of words related to the English word "menstruation"
include mental, memory, meditation, mensurate, commensurate,
meter, mother, mana, magnetic, mead, mania, man, and moon.

Calcium Food Source: Blackberries, blackcurrants, grapes, dates, mulberries, orange, pomegranates, prickly pears, amaranth leaves, bok choy, brussel sprouts, butternut squash, celery, chinese broccoli, french beans, kale, okra, parsnip, spirulina, swiss chard, turnip, brazil nuts, almond, oats, pistachios, sesame seeds, wheat (durum and hard) soy beans (edamame), white beans, winged beans, navy beans, asparagus, barley, basil, zucchini, lemon, tangerine, mustard, greens, thyme, hummus, eggplant, black beans, lentils, tofu, parsley, lima beans, pinto beans, garlic, coriander, winter squash, figs, apricots, prunes, watercress, cabbage, kelp, spinach, and tempeh.

CHLORIDE (Cl) – Trace Mineral Two types: Sodium and Calcium

When salt in the body increases, the combined phenomena of low blood pressure and weakness are symptoms of a chloride deficiency. When this chloride mineral drops down, the body experience loss of potassium via the urine. This is a dangerous condition causing the blood pH level to become elevated. Affected person can lose the ability to control muscle function, leading to problems with breathing, swallowing and even death.

Chloride Food Sources: Kelp, and tomatoes.

CHROMIUM (Cr) – Trace Mineral

Assist absorption our body to absorb and stabilizes energy needed throughout the day. Sufficient quantities can make many large biological molecules that help us survive. It can also help increase muscle mass while reducing fat mass in our bodies. But it is often difficult to get enough chromium in our diets. People who exercise frequently have especially high demands for this element.

Chromium Food Source: Broccoli, brewer's yeast, whole wheat, rye, tomato, spinach, sweet potatoes with skin, dried beans, onion, garlic, barley, oats, green beans, romaine lettuce, wild yam, nettle, catnip, oat straw, licorice, horsetail, yarrow, red clover and sarsaparilla, and brown rice.

Only the rhesus macaque (macaca mulatta—old world monkey) at a 29-day cycle is close to the human menstrual cycle.

COBALT (Co) – Trace Mineral

Without cobalt, Vitamin B-12 could not exist. The body uses this vitamin for numerous of purposes like digestion and nerve function where B12 deficiency can also cause nerve cells to form incorrectly, resulting in irreversible nerve damage. This situation is characterized by symptoms such as delusions, eye disorders, dizziness, confusion, and memory loss. B-12 is necessary for the normal formation of all cells, especially red blood cells. Strict vegetarians are at risk of B-12 deficiency because vegetables do not contain this important vitamin. B-12 can be found in animal sources such as red meat, fish, eggs, cheese, and milk. Alternatively, you can get plenty of vitamin B-12 from most multi-vitamin supplements.

Cobalt Food Sources: Green leafy vegetables as spinach and kale, nuts, oat cereals, cayenne pepper, dandelion, and echinacea.

COPPER (Cu) – Trace Mineral

Is a necessary part of the body's ability to produce hemoglobin. It also works together with iron in the formation of red blood cells. Without copper, the body could not complete the process of building the bones that make up the skeletal system. When the body experiences this rare deficiency, it also means a deficiency in iron. Symptoms like anemia, anorexia nervosa, starvation and kidney problems are taken account from this.

Copper Food Source: Avocado, kiwi, blackberries, dates, guava, lychee, mango, passionfruit, pomegranate, amaranth leaves, artichoke, french beans, kale, lima beans, parsnip, peas, potatoes, pumpkin, spirulina, winter squash, celery, garlic, radishes, mushrooms, pecans, cocoa, prunes, bananas, cherries, raisins, barley, artichokes, sweet potatoes, swiss chard, taro,,brazil nuts, buckwheat, cashews, chestnuts, filberts/hazelnuts, oats, sunflower seeds, walnuts, Wheat/durum and hard red, adzuki beans, kidney beans, white beans, dried prunes, black beans, black eye peas, fava beans soy beans/ edamame, lima beans, navy beans, pigeon beans, pinto beans, and winged beans.

Scholars suggest that pre-modern men and women learned to think numerically by recognizing relationships between groups of numbers that were also units of time measured through menstrual rites.

GERANIUM (GE) – Trace Mineral

Helps in healthy functioning of the immune system and aids the body in cleansing toxins and wound healing. It also helps to fight pain. One of its main functions is to stimulate cells to increase their intake of oxygen and provide the body more energy.

Geranium Food Sources: Wheat, bran, legumes, tomato juice, broccoli, celery, garlic, onions, shitake mushrooms, rhubarb, sauerkraut, aloe vera, comfrey chlorella, and ginseng.

IODINE (I) – Trace Mineral

Seventy-five percent of this mineral makes its way to the thyroid gland then joins up with two important hormones—triiodothyronine and thyroxin. Every part of the body requires these hormones to produce energy. These hormones determine how fast and how efficiently the body is able to burn calories. This can make the amount of fat in the blood supply to increase, thyroid gland can become enlarged, and hoarseness can develop in the throat and in children, possibly causing mental retardation.

Iodine Food Sources: Kelp, navy beans, cranberries, iodized salt, strawberries, kombu, and potatoes.

IRON (Fe) Trace Mineral

It is easy to get enough iron if we can maintain a balance diet. But ironically, iron deficiency anemia is the most common nutritional disease in the world affecting at least five million people. Iron is crucial element to sustain healthy immune system, digestion, and hemoglobin which is carrier of oxygen to our body. In addition, certain chemicals in our brain are controlled by the presence or absence of iron. Studies have shown that women who do not get sufficient amounts of iron may suffer anovulation (lack of ovulation) and possibly poor egg health, which can inhibit pregnancy at a rate 60% higher than those with sufficient iron stores in their blood.

Iron Food Source: Blackberries, avocado, boysenberries, blackcurrant, breadfruits, cherries, dates, figs grapes, kiwi, lemon, loganberries, lychee, mulberries, passion fruit, persimmon, pomegranate, raspberry, strawberry, watermelon, peas, potatoes, pumpkin seeds, amaranth leave, bok choy, brussel sprout, leeks, kale, swiss chard, spirulina, lima beans, french beans, butternut squash, coconut, pine nuts, wheat (duram and hard), spelts, rye, cashews, adzumi beans, black beans, pinto beans, white beans, navy beans, navy beans, pigeon peas, split peas, winged beans, mung beans, kidney beans, garbanzo beans, black eye peas, blueberries, strawberries, bananas, mango, garlic, tomatoes, celery, burdock, Echinacea, yarrow, chickweed, red clover, sunflower seeds, pumpkin seeds, molasses, cashews, peanuts, and paprika.

MAGNESIUM (Mg) – Major Mineral

Magnesium plays a significant role in about 300 biochemical processes that take place inside the body. This is needed to properly develop and maintain the skeletal system and essential to the body's ability to absorb calcium. Magnesium deficiency can lead a person to experience heart disease, diabetes and osteoporosis. It can help to keep muscles and mind relaxed. Migraine, numbness, muscle cramps, anxiety problem, and changes in personality can be symptoms of lacking sufficient magnesium.

Magnesium Food Source: Lemon, zucchini, tangerine, nectarines, artichokes, plums, whole wheat bread, coconut milk, cranberries, apricots, honeydew, papaya, prunes, cauliflower, garlic, asparagus, barley, basil, peppers, pepper, brussel sprouts, buckwheat, cashews, chili peppers, coriander, dill, fennel, figs, flaxseed, onions, hazelnuts, leeks, lima beans, millet, shiitake mushrooms, rosemary, mustard greens, navy beans, parsley, pinto beans, rye, sesame seeds, soy sauce, soy beans, summer squash, winter squash, sunflower seeds, swiss chard, thyme, tempeh, turnip greens, a shake, chocolate, chia seeds, spirulina, quinoa, watermelon, dates, guava, lima beans, avocado, blackberries, raspberries, pinto beans, okra, oats, peanuts, cantaloupe, peach, pineapple, grapefruit, mango, dill, basil, rosemary, spearmint, and peppermint.

Menstrual blood was thought to cure warts, birthmarks, gout, goiters, hemorrhoids, epilepsy, worms, leprosy, and headaches. It was also used in love, could ward off demons, and was occasionally used as an offering to a god. The first napkin worn by a virgin was thought to be a cure for the plague. Menstrual blood was thought to cure warts, birthmarks, gout, goiters, hemorrhoids, epilepsy, worms, leprosy, and headaches.

MANGANESE (Mn) – Trace Mineral

Manganese is not only anti- but also responsible in developing bones, metabolic process, and reproduction function. A manganese deficiency can cause painful joints, osteoporosis, memory loss and diabetes.

Manganese Food Source: Blackberries, blueberries, raspberries, avocado, blackcurrant, guava, grapefruit, gooseberries, loganberries, pineapples, pomegranate, strawberries, dates, cranberries, boysenberries, peas, potatoes, spirulina, kale, leeks, lima beans, parsnip, butternut squash, sweet potato, swiss chard, buckwheat, coconut, pecans, macadamia nuts, pine nuts, almonds, hazelnuts, grapes, kiwi, garlic, mustard greens, cloves, turmeric, leeks, cucumber, peppermint, coconuts, bananas, molasses, beet root, watercress, lettuce, blackberries, soy beans, white beans, winged beans, pigeon beans, garbanzo beans, potatoes, brussel sprouts, French beans, taro, brazil nuts, cashews, amaranth leaves, black tea, saffron, and ginger.

MOLYBDENUM (Mo) – Trace Mineral

Is important in helping our cells grow. Small amount of molybdenum promotes healthy teeth and rand gum problems, lack of oxygen in the blood, loss of appetite and weight.

Molybdenum Food Sources: Navy beans, lentils, black eye peas, split peas, lima beans, kidney beans, almonds, chestnuts, peanuts, cashews, soybeans, black beans, chickpeas, green leafy vegetables, seeds, green beans, and tomatoes.

NICKEL (Ni) – Trace Mineral

It helps activate certain enzymes and involved in the activity of hormones and cell membrane. Low blood levels of nickel are observed in people with vitamin B6 deficiency, cirrhosis of the liver, and kidney failure. Elevated blood levels of nickel, on the other hand, are associated with the development of cancer, heart attack, thyroid disorders, psoriasis and eczema. This suggests the need of balance intake to avoid the opposite adverse results.

Nickel Food Source: Cocoa, cashews, kidney beans, spinach, dried apricot, figs, and prunes, soybeans (edamame), chick peas/garbanzo beans, lentils, yellow peas, mung beans, peanuts, hazelnuts, almonds, walnuts, oat bran, buckwheat, wheat, and millet.

PHOSPHORUS (P) – Major Mineral

Phosphorus maintains healthy blood sugar levels. Phosphorus is also found in substantial amounts in the nervous system. Phosphorus deficiency can occur in those who regularly take antacids, fatigued and weakness are symptoms of mild phosphate deficiency. However, too much intake from processed foods, soft drinks, and meats may lead to osteoporosis.

Phosphorus Food Source: Bananas, apples, oranges, watermelon, strawberries, avocado, blueberries, broccoli, almonds, cucumber, honey, pears, pineapple, cantaloupe, celery, oatmeal, cherries, grapefruit, brown rice, tomatoes, mushrooms, potatoes, salad, sweet potato, green beans, butternut squash, peanuts, pumpkin seeds, quinoa, a mango, mango, pecans, raisins, spinach, spirulina, walnuts, oats, cabbage, beets, garbanzo beans, tofu, kiwi, lentils, pomegranate, kale, black beans, coconut, dates, kidney beans, hummus, eggplant, lemon, zucchini, tangerine, nectarines, artichokes, plums, cranberries, apricots, honeydew, papaya, prunes, prune juice, cauliflower, garlic, brazil nuts, sunflower seeds, spelt, rye, pine nuts, black eye peas, kidney beans, lima beans, pinto beans, garbanzo beans, navy beans, white beans, and parsley.

POTASSIUM (K) – Major Mineral

Intake of sodium should be balanced to avoid heart disease and maintaining positive and negative ions in our body fluids and tissues. Sodium aids in preventing heat prostration or sunstroke.

Potassium: Avocado, blackcurrants, bananas, breadfruit, cherimoya, cherries, Chinese pear, grapefruit, dates, guava, kiwi, lychee, papaya, passion fruit, pomegranate, prickly pear, watermelon, swiss chard, sweet potatoes, garlic, spirulina, pumpkin, parsnip, lima beans, French beans, butternut squash, bok choy, bamboo shoots, amaranth leaves, almonds, buckwheat, chestnuts, coconut, oats, pistachios, pumpkin seeds, sunflower seeds, rye, wheat (durum, hard), adzuki beans, pinto beans, lima beans, soy beans, white beans, kidney beans, swiss chard, kale, zucchini, spinach, mushroom, Brussel sprouts, green beans, asparagus, thyme, parsley, basil, black beans, lemons, cabbage, beets, mustard greens, cashews, hazelnuts, cucumber, and turnip greens.

SELENIUM (Se) – Trace Mineral

Selenium has cancer-fighting potential and antioxidant properties. It protects against the formation of free radicals—unstable oxygen molecules caused by muscle movement, metabolism, and inhalation of smoke and pollution. I protects eggs and sperm from free radicals. Free radicals can cause chromosomal damage known to be a cause of miscarriages and birth defects. Selenium is also necessary for the creation of sperm. In studies of men with low sperm counts, they have been found to have low levels of selenium.

Selenium Food Source: Brazil nuts, bananas, breadfruit, guava, lychee, mango, passion fruit, pomegranate, watermelon, lima beans, peas, parsnip, mushrooms (shitake, crimini and button), spirulina, French beans, asparagus, Brussel sprouts, mung beans, navy beans, pigeon beans, plantains, spinach, black eye peas, fava beans, wheat, barley, brown rice, oats, garlic, ginger, parsley, garlic, onions, lentils, brown rice, brazil nuts, broccoli, grapefruit, and amaranth.

SILICON (Si) – Major Mineral

This element is essential in the functioning of nerve cells and tissues because it controls the transmission of nerve impulses. It is also called "beauty mineral," because it protects the eyes and skin and essential for the growth of our teeth, nails, and hair. For diseases like tuberculosis, irritations in the mucous membranes, and skin disorders—silicon contributes in the healing process.

Silicon Food Source: Romaine lettuce, almonds, flaxseeds, millet, almonds, peanuts, tomato, nopal cactus, radish, spinach, marjoram, horsetail, hemp leaves, cucumber, grapes, raisins, oranges, apples, burdock root, barley, beets, brown rice, oats, soy beans, bell peppers, bananas, whole wheat, and alfalfa, blue cohosh, comfrey, leafy green vegetables, chickweed, dandelion, red raspberry, stinging nettles, red peppers, celery, beets, potatoes, carrots, cornsilk, and red lentils.

Eighty-one percent of women say they've experienced dysmenorrhea (painful cramps). This occurs because the prostaglandin hormone causes the uterus to cramp, causing the abdomen to spasm.

SODIUM (Na) – Major Mineral

Sodium is important in the distribution of water in the body. It helps maintain fluid volume in the vessels and tissues.

Sodium Food Source: Guava, strawberry, passion fruit, amaranth leaves, coconut, winged beans, artichoke, beetroot, broccoli, bok choy, Brussel sprouts, celery, fennel, kale, spirulina, spaghetti squash, sweet potato, swiss chard, pumpkin seeds, quinoa, spelt, winged beans, tamarinds, honeydew, cantaloupe, mulberries, kumquats, and strawberries.

SULFUR (S) – Major Mineral

This essential element can easily be found in almost all food we eat. Sulfur defends the body's cells from environmental hazards such as air pollution and radiation. In addition, sulfur helps our liver function correctly; it digests food and turns it into energy. It can help to slow the aging process and extend the life span in humans. It keeps skin supple and elastic as well.

Sulfur Food Source: garlic, lettuce, cabbage, brussel sprouts, broccoli, cauliflower, cabbage, kale, turnips, bok choy, and kohlrabi, walnuts, almonds, sesame seeds, sunflower seeds, coconut, banana, watermelon, mustard greens, water cress, kale, garlic, onions, dried beans, asparagus, leeks, peas, chives, avocado, peanuts, pistachios, and wheat germ.

TIN (Sn) – Trace Mineral

Primarily supports function of the adrenal gland. Psychological benefits includes decreased depression and fatigue, an increase in positive mood, and general well-being, and energy. Some test subjects also experienced improvements in general occurrences of pain, skin problems, and digestion. There was also a noticeable decrease in headaches, asthma, and insomnia for some.

Tin Food Source: Kelp, figs, dog grass, juniper, bilberry, milk thistle, dulse, lady slipper, althea, valerian, Irish moss, nettle, barberry, yarrow, blessed thistle, yellow dock, licorice, devils claw, pennyroyal, and senna. Found in nearly all fruits and vegetables.

A young woman can get her first period anywhere between 10 and 16 years of age. Delayed onset of menstruation is rare, but if a girl has not started by the age of 16, she should see a gynecologist. In the United States, 97.5% of women have begun their menstrual cycles by the age 16.

VANADIUM (V) – Trace Mineral

There may be some potential health benefits provided by vanadium for those with bipolar disorder. Researchers believe when people are in the manic state of bipolar disorder their vanadium levels are significantly elevated, which means a diet reducing vanadium intake can benefit those with bipolar disorder.

Vanadium Food Source: Mushrooms, parsley, dill weed, buckwheat, green beans, corn, carrots, radishes, oats, cabbage, garlic, tomatoes, onions, olives, snap beans, black pepper.

ZINC (Zn) – Trace Mineral

Sixty-seven percent of the U.S. population suffers from zinc deficiency. Sufficient amount ensure the immune system remains healthy and can fight off disease. It helps produce and activate T-lymphocytes; one type of white blood cell the body uses to help fight infection. It can hamper sexual function and capability, impotence, lethargy, loss of appetite and diminished immune capability. In women, zinc works with more than 300 enzymes to keep the body working well. Without it, your cells can not divide properly; your estrogen and progesterone levels can get out of balance and your reproductive system may not fully function. Low levels of zinc have been directly linked to miscarriage in the initial stages of a pregnancy, according to The Centers for Disease Control's Assisted Reproductive Technology Report.

In men, zinc is considered one of the most important trace minerals for male fertility; increasing zinc levels in infertile men has been shown to boost sperm levels, and; improve the form, function, and quality of male sperm.

Scholars debate the existence of menstrual synchronicity (a.k.a. the McClintock effect or dormitory effect), a theory that suggests that women who live in close proximity to each other develop synchronized periods.

Zinc Food Source: Bananas, apples, oranges, wine, watermelon, strawberry, avocado, blueberries, broccoli, almonds, cucumber, pears, pineapple, cantaloupe, peaches, celery, cherries, grapefruit, brown rice, tomatoes, mushrooms, potatoes, sweet potato, nuts, orange juice, green beans, tuna, skim milk, fish, butternut squash, peanuts, pumpkin seeds, quinoa, mango, pecans, raisins, spinach, spirulina, walnuts, oats, cabbage, beets, garbanzo beans, tofu, kiwi, lentils, pomegranate, kale, black beans, coconut, dates, kidney beans, hummus, eggplant, lemon, zucchini, tangerine, nectarines, artichokes, plums, cranberries, apricots, honeydew, papaya, prunes, cauliflower, garlic, asparagus, barley, basil, brussel sprouts, buckwheat, cashews, chili peppers, coriander, dill, fennel, figs, flaxseed, tea, onions, yams, hazelnuts, leeks, lima beans, millet, shiitake mushrooms, rosemary, mustard greens, navy beans, parsley, pinto beans, rye, sesame seeds, soybeans, summer squash, winter squash, sunflower seeds, swiss chard, thyme, tempeh, turnip greens, chia seeds, brewer's yeast, and pecans."

In many cultures, a fetus was thought to be formed in the womb by clotting menstrual blood.

ELECTROLYTES

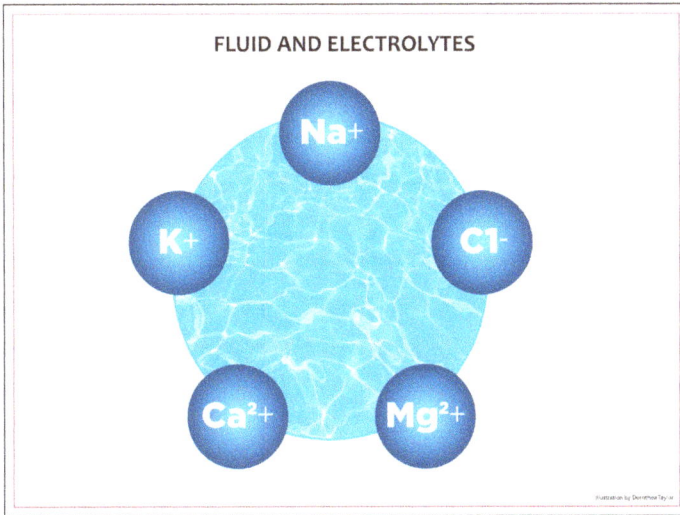

FLUID AND ELECTROLYTES

"Electrolyte is a "medical/scientific" term for salts, specifically ions. Electrolytes are salts in the body that conduct electricity and are found in the tissue, and body fluids. For example, your body fluids – blood, plasma, and interstitial fluid (fluid between cells) – are like seawater and have a high concentration of **sodium chloride** (table salt, or NaCl). The term electrolyte means this ion is electrically charged and moves to either a **negative (cathode)** or **positive (anode) electrode**:
  • ions that move to the cathode (**cations**) are positively charged.
  • ions that move to the anode (**anions**) are negatively charged.

In some parts of India, a woman indicates she is menstruating by wearing a handkerchief around her neck stained with her menstrual blood.

For instance, the electrolytes in sodium chloride (NaCl) are:
- **sodium ion** (Na+) - cation
- **chloride ion** (Cl-) – anion

Sodium (Na+) is concentrated in the extracellular fluid between tissue cells and potassium (K+) is concentrated in the intracellular fluid within the blood vessels. Proper balance is essential for muscle coordination, heart function, fluid absorption and excretion, nerve function, and concentration.

As for your body, the major electrolytes are as follows:
1. sodium (Na+)
2. potassium (K+) 3. chloride (Cl-)
4. calcium (Ca2+)
5. magnesium (Mg2+)
6. bicarbonate (HCO3-)
7. phosphate (PO42-)
8. sulfate (SO42-)

The **kidneys regulate fluid absorption and excretion** and maintain a narrow range of electrolyte fluctuation. Normally, sodium and potassium are filtered and excreted in the urine and feces according to the body's needs. When the body has too much or too little sodium or potassium, caused by poor diet, dehydration, medication, and/or disease, results in an imbalance.

Fluids in the body contain water and a variety of dissolved chemicals. Some of these chemicals exist in the form of compounds called electrolytes. Electrolytes are needed for metabolism, for movement of fluids, and normal cellular activities.

ELECTROLYTE LEVELS ARE CONTROLLED BY HORMONES

Adrenals produce hormones

The adrenal glands are located on the top of each kidney. The adrenals produce about 50 hormones, including adrenaline, epinephrine, and norepinephrine, which are responsible for our fight or flight response. They also **produce hormones** that allow our muscles to grow and our carbohydrates and **electrolytes to be metabolized**. About two-thirds of the body's fluid is **intracellular** (located inside cells). The other third is **extracellular** (located outside cells). Extracellular fluid contains substantial amounts of sodium, but only lesser amounts of potassium Intracellular fluids contain the opposite. Extracellular fluids supply the cells with nutrients and other substances needed for cellular function. But, before the cell can utilize these substances, they must be transported through the cell membrane.

Both the amount of water and the concentration of electrolytes are important to bodily functions. When the body is "in fluid balance" it means that the various body compartments (cells, tissues, organs) contain the required number of fluids to carry out normal bodily functions. Fluid balance and electrolyte balance are inseparable. In a healthy individual, the volume of fluid in each compartment remains stable.

ELECTROLYTES SERVE THREE GENERAL FUNCTIONS

1. Electrolytes are needed for **normal metabolism**. Many electrolytes are essential minerals, some organic and some inorganic. Acids, bases, and salts are electrolytes. They are called electrolytes because they can conduct electric currents. Acids (proton donors) and bases (proton acceptors) react to one another to form salts in the body.

2. Electrolytes are needed for **proper fluid movement** between compartments (from cell to cell, tissue to tissue, and organ to organ). The walls of compartments are semipermeable. Through osmosis, fluids are in constant movement from one compartment to another within fractions of a second. The concentration (and the nature) of the solutes in the fluids are a major determinant of fluid balance.

3. Electrolytes help **maintain the acid-base (Alkalinity) balance** required for normal cellular activities. In a healthy person pH is between **6.4 and 7.00**.

Homeostasis of this range is essential to survival and depends on three major mechanisms in the body: 1) Buffer systems, which work within fractions of a second to prevent drastic changes in body fluid pH; 2) Respirations, which can increase or decrease pH levels within 1-3 minutes; and 3) Kidney excretions.

ELECTROLYTE LOSS

Loss of Electrolytes can occur through long term laxative use and use of diuretic medications. It can also result from vomiting, diarrhea and any form of water loss that results in dehydration. Sodium can also be lost through excessive perspiration and burns. Potassium can also be lost through high sodium intake and kidney disease. The specific chemical elements of electrolytes and consequences from their loss are described below.

CHEMICAL ELEMENTS OF ELECTROLYTES

The chemical elements of electrolytes are **sodium, chloride, potassium, calcium, phosphate,** and **magnesium**. Loss of electrolytes can have profound consequences for the body. In severe dehydration, the loss of electrolytes can result in **circulatory problems** such as tachycardia (rapid heartbeat) and problems with the nervous system such as **loss of consciousness**.

Sodium is necessary for nerve impulse transmission, muscular contraction and fluid and electrolyte balance. Sodium level in the blood is controlled by aldosterone. Hyponatremia, a lower than normal blood sodium level, is characterized by muscular weakness, headache, hypotension, tachycardia, and circulatory shock. Severe hyponatremia can result in mental confusion, stupor, and coma.

Chloride can easily diffuse between extracellular and intracellular compartments. This makes chloride important in regulating osmotic pressure differences between compartments. Chloride level is indirectly controlled by aldosterone. Hypochloremia, an abnormally low level of chloride in the blood, results in muscle spasms, alkalosis, depressed respirations, and coma.

Potassium helps to maintain fluid volume in cells and **regulates pH**. Potassium has a vital role in nerve impulse conduction and muscle contraction. Potassium level is controlled by aldosterone. Hypokalemia, loss of potassium, results in cramps and fatigue, flaccid paralysis, mental confusion, increased urine output, shallow respirations, and changes in the electrocardiogram.

Calcium and **Phosphate** are stored in the **bones and teeth** and released when needed. Calcium and phosphate are structural components of bones and teeth. Calcium required for blood clotting, chemical transmitter release, muscle contraction and normal heartbeat. Phosphate is necessary for the formation of nucleic acids, the synthesis of high energy compounds and buffering reactions. Calcium and phosphate levels in the blood are regulated by several hormones.

Magnesium is important for the sodium-potassium pump which controls the volume of the cells. Without the function of this pump, most cells of the body would swell until they burst. The pump activates enzyme systems needed to produce cellular energy. It is the basis of nerve function to transmit signals throughout the nervous system. Magnesium levels are regulated by aldosterone. Hypomagnesemia, magnesium loss, results in increased neuromuscular and nervous system irritability leading to tremor, tetany, and convulsions. Loss of magnesium through diuretic use can result in cardiac arrhythmias.

Electrolytes are important because they are what your cells (especially nerve, heart, muscle) use to maintain voltages across their cell membranes and to carry electrical impulses (nerve impulses, muscle contractions) across themselves and to other cells. Your kidneys work to keep the electrolyte concentrations in your blood constant despite changes in your body. For example, when you exercise heavily, you lose electrolytes in your sweat, particularly sodium and potassium. These electrolytes must be replaced to keep the electrolyte concentrations of your body fluids constant."

Up until the age of about 18, irregular periods are quite common because the body is still working on perfecting the system.

AMINO ACIDS

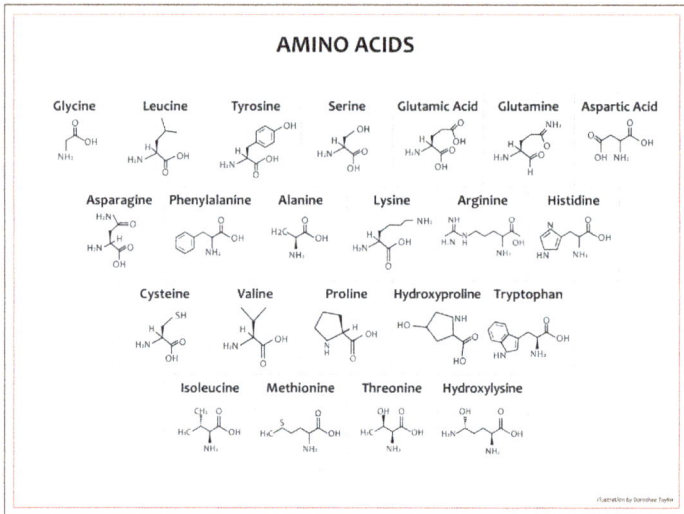

AMINO ACIDS

According to Med Line Plus Trusted Health Information for You, amino acids are organic compounds that combine to form proteins. Amino acids and proteins are the building blocks of life. Twenty percent of the human body is made up of protein. Protein plays a crucial role in almost all biological processes and amino acids are the building blocks of it.

A sizable proportion of our cells, muscles and tissue is made up of amino acids, meaning they conduct many important bodily functions, such as giving cells their structure. They also play a key role in the transport and the storage of nutrients. Amino acids have an influence on the function of organs, glands, tendons, and arteries. They are furthermore essential for healing wounds and repairing tissue, especially in the muscles, bones, skin and hair as well as for the removal of all kinds of waste deposits produced in connection with the metabolism.

When proteins are digested or broken down, amino acids are left. The human body uses amino acids to make proteins to help the body:

- Break down food
- Grow
- Repair body tissue
- Perform many other body functions

Amino acids can also be used as a source of energy by the body.
Amino acids are classified into three groups:

- Essential amino acids
- Nonessential amino acids
- Conditional amino acid

Nine Essential amino acids

- Essential amino acids cannot be made by the body. As a result, they must come from food.
- The nine essential amino acids are: histidine, isoleucine, leucine, lysine, methionine, phenylalanine, threonine, tryptophan, and valine.

Four Nonessential amino acids

- "Nonessential" means that our bodies produce an amino acid, even if we do not get it from the food we eat.
- They include: alanine, asparagine, aspartic acid, and glutamic acid.

Eight Conditional amino acids

- Conditional amino acids are usually not essential, except in times of illness and stress.
- They include: arginine, cysteine, glutamine, tyrosine, glycine, ornithine, proline, and serine.

You do not need to eat essential and nonessential amino acids at every meal but getting a balance of them over the whole day is important.

GOOD PLANT-BASED SOURCES FOR
THE NINE ESSENTIAL AMINO ACIDS

Leucine

seaweed, pumpkin, peas and pea protein, whole grain rice, sesame seeds, watercress, turnip greens, soy, sunflower seeds, kidney beans, figs, avocados, raisins, dates, apples, blueberries, olives and even bananas. Do not limit yourself to one food of these choices, and aim for a serving of either seaweed, leafy greens, hemp seeds, chia seeds, grains, legumes, seeds, or beans at each meal to be sure you get enough high-quality plant protein.

Isoleucine

rye, soy, cashews, almonds, oats, lentils, beans, brown rice, cabbage, hemp seeds, chia seeds, spinach, pumpkin, pumpkin seeds, sunflower seeds, sesame seeds, cranberries, quinoa, blueberries, apples, and kiwis.

Lysine

beans (the best), watercress, hemp seeds, chia seeds, spirulina, parsley, avocados, soy protein, almonds, cashews, and some legumes with lentils and chickpeas being two of the best.

Methionine

sunflower seed butter and sunflower seeds, hemp seeds, chia seeds, Brazil nuts, oats, seaweed, wheat, figs, whole grain rice, beans, legumes, onions, cacao, and raisins.

Phenylalanine

spirulina and other seaweed, pumpkin, beans, rice, avocado, almonds, peanuts, quinoa, figs, raisins, leafy greens, most berries, olives, and seeds.

Threonine

watercress and spirulina (which even exceed meat), pumpkin, leafy greens, hemp seeds, chia seeds, soybeans, sesame seeds, sunflower seeds and sunflower butter, almonds, avocados, figs, raisins, quinoa, and wheat. Sprouted grains are also excellent sources of this amino acid as well.

Tryptophan

oats and oat bran, seaweed, hemp seeds, chia seeds, spinach, watercress, soybeans, pumpkin, sweet potatoes, parsley, beans, beats, asparagus, mushrooms, all lettuces, leafy greens, beans, avocado, figs, winter squash, celery, peppers, carrots, chickpeas, onions, apples, oranges, bananas, quinoa, lentils, and peas.

Valine

beans, spinach, legumes, broccoli, sesame seeds, hemp seeds, chia seeds, soy, peanuts, whole grains, figs, avocado, apples, sprouted grains and seeds, blueberries, cranberries, oranges, and apricots.

Histidine

rice, wheat, rye, seaweed, beans, legumes, cantaloupe, hemp seeds, chia seeds, buckwheat, potatoes, cauliflower, and corn.

GOOD PLANT-BASED SOURCES FOR THE EIGHT CONDITIONAL AMINO ACIDS

Moringa Oleifera is a storehouse of important nutrients and is used both for its nutritional and therapeutic properties. Apart from storing important levels of vitamins and minerals, **it also carries all the amino acids needed for the growth and maintenance of a healthy body.**

In 2007, the World Health Organization (WHO) also documented the fact that the amino acid contents of moringa leaf are higher than required amounts for healthy child's growth.

Arginine

cauliflower, apricot, mango, avocado, bamboo shoot, zucchini, navy beans, squash, green beans, sweet potatoes, azuki bens, asparagus, rapini, guava, kidney beans, black beans, carrot, spinach, kale, lotus root, white potato, bok choy, corn, turnip greens, leek, mung bean, lima beans, okra, cowpeas, watercress, lentils, swiss chard, chestnuts, brussel sprouts, barley, soybeans, peas, water spinach, seaweed (dried), chick peas, broccoli, and quinoa.

Cysteine

nuts, seeds, soy products, legumes, oatmeal, carrots, mushrooms, couscous, rice, wheat products, (seitan/pasta), brussels sprouts, broccoli, onions and red bell peppers.

Glutamine

spinach, cabbage, parsley, beets, black beans, kidney beans, peas, lentils, oats, wheat germ, quinoa, millet, brown rice, almonds, pistachios, walnuts, pumpkin seeds, sunflower seeds, peanuts, and peanut butter.

Tyrosine

soy products, peanuts, almonds, avocados, spinach, bananas, milk, cheese, yogurt, cottage cheese, lima beans, pumpkin seeds, and sesame seeds.

Glycine

peanuts, granola, seaweed, carob seeds, watercress, asparagus, cabbage, tofu, spinach, beets, sweet potatoes, carrots, pear, apple, banana, carrots whole grains, sunflower, sesame and pumpkin seeds, cashews, pistachios, and legumes.

Ornithine

is predominantly found in meat, fish, dairy, and eggs.

Proline

watercress, alfalfa sprouts, cucumber, cabbage, chives, gelatin, soy protein, cabbage, asparagus, mushrooms, sunflower seeds and seaweed.

Serine

Soy protein, soy meal, hemp seed, pumpkin seed, butternuts, pistachios, peanuts, black walnuts, fenugreek seed, sesame seeds, cashew nuts, sunflower seeds, chia seeds, chickpeas, soy beans, poppy seeds, fennel seeds, oat bran, pine nuts, lupin beans, mustard seeds, hazel nuts, raw buckwheat, wheat bran, brazil nuts, edamame, rice bran, pili nuts, pinto beans, kidney beans, goji berries, lentil sprouts, pink beans, black beans, navy beans, pecans, chili peppers, lima beans, macadamia nuts, lentils, black pepper, adzuki beans, peas, fava beans, mung beans, wheat sprouts, pigeon peas, oatmeal, oregano, beechnuts, spirulina, pea sprouts, laver, turmeric, clove, soba, lotus seeds, ground ginger, wild rice, broad beans, millet, mustard, cinnamon, garlic, green peas, tef, couscous, quinoa, buckwheat, dill weed, sweet corn, chives, peppermint, bulgar, parsley, rosemary, spearmint, broccoli, avocado, shallots, asparagus, spinach, jackfruit, basil, kelp, leeks, rapini, pearl barley, white mushrooms, welsh onions, cauliflower, potatoes, apricot, raw sweet potato, carambola, chestnuts, hearts of palm, hot chili pepper, yam, and wakame.

GOOD PLANT-BASED SOURCES
FOUR NONESSENTIAL AMINO ACIDS

Alanine

watercress, soy, beans, asparagus, spinach, seeds of watermelon, lentils, cauliflower, pumpkin seeds, peanuts, broad beans, corn, sunflower seeds and green peas.

Asparagine

asparagus, potatoes, legumes, nuts, seeds, soy, almonds, whole grains, and oat.

Aspartic acid

avocado, asparagus, Molasses, nectarines, legumes, peanuts, soy, chickpeas, lentils, oats, corn, pistachios, walnuts, chestnuts, almonds, sesame seeds, sunflower seeds, pine nuts, spinach, pumpkins, potatoes, carrots, eggplants, peppers, celery, lettuce, chicory, garlic, onions, apricots, oranges, pears, papaya, bananas, grapes, mango, figs, apples, and currants.

Glutamic acid

Beans, broccoli, parsley, spinach, soy, whole grains, rice, bread, durum wheat, raw spinach, raw parsley, kidney beans, soybeans, collard greens, kale, lettuce, green and white asparagus, and red cabbage.

22 AMINO ACIDS
(INCLUDING 3-LETTER AND 1-LETTER IDENTIFIERS)

1. Alanine (Ala) (A) — Nonessential
2. Arginine (Arg) (R) — Nonessential
3. Asparagine (Asn) (N) — Nonessential
4. Aspartic acid (Asp) (D) — Nonessential
5. Cysteine (Cys) (C) – Nonessential
6. Cystine (Cys) (C) — Nonessential
7. Glutamine (Gln) (Q) – Nonessential
8. Glutamic acid (Glu) (E) — Nonessential
9. Glycine (Gly) (G) — Nonessential
10. Histidine (His) (H) – Nonessential
11. Hydroxyproline (Hyp) (H) – Nonessential

12. Isoleucine (Ile) (I) – Essential
13. Leucine (Leu) (L) – Essential
14. Lysine (Lys) (K) – Essential
15. Methionine (Met) (M) – Essential
16. Phenylalanine (Phe) (F) – Essential
17. Proline (Pro) (P) – Nonessential
18. Serine (Ser) (S) – Nonessential
19. Threonine (Thr) (T) – Essential
20. Tryptophan (Trp) (W) – Essential
21. Tyrosine (Tyr) (Y) – Nonessential
22. Valine (Val) (V) – Essential

1. ALANINE (Non-Essential Amino Acid)

Is an important source of energy for muscle tissue, the brain and central nervous system; strengthens the immune system by producing antibodies; helps in the metabolism of sugars and organic acids.

2. ARGININE (Non-Essential Amino Acid)

It improves immune responses to bacteria, viruses, and tumor cells, promotes wound healing and regeneration of the liver, causes the release of growth hormones, considered crucial for optimal muscle growth and tissue repair. Arginine stimulates the growth of new bone and tendon cells.

3. ASPARAGINE (Non-Essential Amino Acid)

On intracellular function, Asparagine, Glutamine and Serine are vital for energy and smooth function of brain reactions; contribute to the formation of proteins, muscles, neurotransmitters, antibodies, and receptors. Asparagine is an important transporter of nitrogen; foundation of carbohydrate metabolism; and improves recovery after surgery or trauma by hastening wound.

4. ASPARTIC ACID (Non-Essential Amino Acid)

Aspartic Acid aids in the expulsion of harmful ammonia from the body. When ammonia enters the circulatory system, it acts as a highly toxic substance which can be harmful to the Central Nervous System.

5. CYSTEINE (Non-Essential Amino Acids)

In addition to protecting the cells from the harmful effects of radiation, [L-Cysteine] protects the liver and brain from damage due to alcohol and cigarette smoke.

6. CYSTINE (Non-Essential Amino Acid)

It functions as an antioxidant and is a powerful aid to the body in protecting against radiation and pollution. It can help slow the aging process, deactivate free radicals, neutralize toxins; and aids in protein synthesis and presents cellular change. It is necessary for the formation of the skin, which aids in the recovery from burns and surgical operations. Hair and skin are made up 10-14% cystine.

7. GLUTAMINE (Non-Essential Amino Acid)

The brain requires a constant supply of energy to think and be alert, Glutamine provides the fuel the brain cells need to think clearly and help combat fatigue.

8. GLUTAMIC ACID (Non-Essential Amino Acid)

Considered to be nature's "brain food" by improving mental capacities, help speed the healing of ulcers; support the digestive track, gives a "lift" from fatigue; control alcoholism, schizophrenia, and the craving for sugar.

9. GLYCINE (Non-Essential Amino Acid)

Helps trigger the release of oxygen to the energy requiring cell-making process; Important in the manufacturing of hormones responsible for a strong immune system.

10. HISTIDINE (Non-Essential Amino Acid)

Is found abundantly in hemoglobin; has been used in the treatment of rheumatoid arthritis, allergic diseases, ulcers, and anemia. A deficiency can cause poor hearing.

11. HYDROXYPROLINE (Non-Essential Amino Acid)

Plays a key role in manufacture of collagen, connective tissue, skin, ligaments, tendons, bones, cartilage and is necessary in Vitamin D assimilation. Vitamin D is essential in proper calcium absorption.

12. ISOLEUCINE (Essential Amino Acid)

Isoleucine stimulates the brain to produce alertness.

13. LEUCINE (Essential Amino Acid)

Leucine stimulates protein synthesis and its importance in protein storage. Both Isoleucine and Leucine provide ingredients for the manufacturing of other essential biochemical components in the body, some of which are utilized for the production of energy—stimulates the upper brain and helps with alertness.

14. LYSINE (Essential Amino Acid)

Lysine is found in the muscle tissue. Soybeans are high in lysine, but rare in other vegetables. Lysine ensures the adequate absorption of calcium; helps form collagen (which makes up bone cartilage and connective tissues), aids in the production of antibodies, hormones, and enzymes. A deficiency may result in tiredness, inability to concentrate, irritability, bloodshot eyes, retarded growth, hair loss, anemia, and reproductive problems.

15. METHIONINE (Essential Amino Acid)

Methionine performs the major roles of being a methyl donor, sulfur donor, and helps lower cholesterol. Methionine is a natural chelating agent for heavy metals, a principle supplier of sulfur that prevents disorders of the hair, skin and nails. It can influence hair follicles and promotes hair growth, increases the liver's production of lecithin and helps reduce cholesterol and liver fat, and regulates the formation of ammonia and creates ammonia-free urine which reduces bladder irritation and promotes kidney health.

16. PHENYLALANINE (Essential Amino Acid)

Phenylalanine, which is highly concentrated in protein foods, is understood to perform as a pain reliever. Phenylalanine is used by the brain to produce norepinephrine, a chemical that transmits signals between nerve cells and the brain. It helps maintain alertness; reduces hunger; acts as an antidepressant, and helps improve memory.

17. PROLINE (Non-Essential Amino Acid)

Essential for proper functioning of joints and tendons, and; helps maintain and strengthen heart muscles.

18. SERINE (Non-Essential Amino Acid)

Is a storage source of glucose by the liver and muscles; helps strengthen the immune system by providing antibodies, and; synthesizes fatty acid sheath around nerve fibers.

19. THREONINE (Essential Amino Acid)

Threonine is the least abundant amino acid, but essential in preventing fat build-up in the liver and assisting digestive and intestinal tracts function more smoothly, assists metabolism and assimilation. Threonine is an important constituent of collagen, elastin, and enamel protein.

20. TRYPTOPHAN (Essential Amino Acid)

Tryptophan is a natural relaxant, helps alleviate insomnia by inducing normal sleep; reduces anxiety and depression, helps in the treatment of migraine headaches and; the immune system by controlling certain intractable pain, helps reduce the risk of artery and heart spasms; works with Lysine in reducing cholesterol levels.

21. TYROSINE (Non-Essential Amino Acid)

Transmits nerve impulses to the brain, helps overcome depression, Improves memory, increases mental alertness, and promotes the healthy functioning of the thyroid, adrenal and pituitary glands. Tyrosine is synthesized in the body from phenylalanine. Like phenylalanine, tyrosine is intimately involved with the important brain neurotransmitters epinephrine, norepinephrine, and dopamine.

22. VALINE (Essential Amino Acid)

Valine promotes mental vigor, muscle coordination and calms emotions.

In German, the word for menstruation is regel, in French it is regle, and in Spanish it is las reglas—which all mean "measure" or "rule" as well as "menstruation" and are cognate [a word of the same origin or root] with "regal," "regalia," and "rex" (king). These terms suggest menstruation is linked to orderliness, ceremony, law, and leadership.

Herbal Support for the Reproductive and Immune Systems

"Plant medicines possess the unique ability of regeneration. They are life supportive, deeply nourishing and can enhance our health in significant ways. We have a natural affinity for plant medicines since we are made of the very same substances. According to Herbologist, Dr. Dorothy Brunslins, herbs are more potent and affective when taking more than one kind as a combination to heal an issue in the body.

There are a large variety of herbs used to support the reproductive system of both men and women. Some are general tonics to support and maintain healthy reproductive function, while others heal and treat specific reproductive problems. Most of these herbs are readily available as whole herbs, powders, or tinctures. Seek the advice of a professional herbalist for dosage information and consult your physician before taking any herbs.

Alfalfa Leaf
This excellent source of nutrients is a digestive aid. It is said to alkalize and detoxify the body. Alfalfa is extremely high in chlorophyll.

Aloe Vera
Is a smooth muscle relaxant that specifically targets the pelvic area and Apana Vayu. It soothes cramps by relaxing muscle tension and spasms.

Some scientists have suggested harvesting stem cells from menstrual blood.

Asafetida

Is known to increase progesterone, a hormone that helps initiate the menstrual process. If your period frequently starts out light, this herb should help to start it on time and maintain more.

Ashwagandha (balances hormones)

Ashwagandha is considered an adaptogen. It also improves physical energy and increases white blood cell formation, thereby increasing immunity and vitality. Ashwagandha stabilizes hormonal balance. It helps to reduce panic attacks, insomnia, and mood swings. It improves memory and cognitive function. Due to an aphrodisiac property, it helps to improve the libido in women during and after menopause. It also has a mild sedative effect on the central nervous system and acts as a muscle relaxant.

Black Cohosh

Famous for its beneficial effects on women's health. The herb is said to provide relief from menstrual problems (including PMS) and may be a natural way to ease menopausal discomforts.

Black Haw (Viburnum prunifolium)

Black Haw have been shown to have a specific action on the uterus, the relaxing action increases circulation to the uterus, allowing for toxin removal that may aid the uterus in healing and overall improvement in uterine health. It is considered the most important uterine antispasmodics. It is extremely effective at reducing uterine contractions, and muscle spasm. Painful menstruation is known as dysmenorrhea, which means "difficult menstruation". Painful menstrual cramps or cramping of the uterus due to threatened miscarriage, miscarriage, or after birth pains, these herbs have the ability to relax smooth muscle, for example: intestines, uterus, air way. Black Haw has a mild sedative action, aiding the body in reducing anxiety, nervous tension, and irritability, while promoting a sense of calm and well-being.

Scholars suggest that marriage rites are an extension of menarchal rites, which may explain why many bridal dresses were historically red. The bride would also walk on a red carpet to the wedding ceremony, wearing a red veil.

Blessed Thistle

Is an old and revered "bitter" herb that is well known for its use in promoting a healthy gastrointestinal system. It is a fine overall tonic that stimulates good digestion, healthy liver, and gallbladder function, and promotes general good health.

Blue Cohosh

Is an important "women's herb" introduced to early American settlers by Native Americans for menstrual problems such as cramps and muscle spasms. It contains an alkaloid called methyl cytosine, which is believed to be antispasmodic. This Native American medicine works primarily to help tone and strengthen the uterus. It also combats painful menstrual flow irregularities by dilating blood vessels in the uterus, allowing for increased circulation in the pelvic area. Modern herbalists still use it to treat women's health problems, as well as bronchitis and rheumatism.

Bupleurum Root

First mentioned in Chinese medical texts as early as A.D. 200, Bupleurum root is considered a deep liver cleanser that helps rid the body of toxins and may ease hepatitis, gallbladder, spleen, and digestive ailments. It also invigorates the circulatory system and promotes health.

Boswellia

An important herb in ancient Ayurvedic medicine -revered for its anti-inflammatory qualities. May relieve muscle pain, joint pain and aches associated with arthritis, gout, carpal tunnel syndrome and osteoarthritis. There are normally no side effects by the steroidal and non-steroidal anti-inflammatory medications usually prescribed for these conditions.

Buchu Leaf

Known to strengthen the urinary system and ease inflammation of the bladder, reduce bloating and excess water weight, alleviate painful, and reduce swelling of the prostate.

In the past, Christian churches refused communion to menstruating women.

Burdock

Helps to rid the body of toxins and clear congestion from the circulatory, lymphatic, respiratory and urinary systems. It is said to soothe the aches and pains of arthritis, alleviate excess water weight and help to keep the skin clear and healthy.

Butcher's Broom Root

Is used to relieve excess fluid in the system and a bloated feeling, varicose veins and swelling brought on by excess water or poor circulation.

Calendula

Its anti-inflammatory and antiseptic qualities have been used for centuries to ease skin infections, ulcerations, diaper rash and varicose veins. The herb is also said to help support the healthy digestion process. Calendula is widely used in cosmetics for its toning and soothing effects.

Cat's Claw

Has become widely recognized as a superior immune stimulant with antioxidant, antiviral and anti-inflammatory qualities. It is said to be a "life-giving" tonic.

Chamomile

Calms Muscle Spasms. One study from England found that drinking chamomile tea raised urine levels of glycine, a compound that calms muscle spasms. Researchers believe this is why chamomile tea could prove to be an effective home remedy for menstrual cramps as well. Soothes Stomachache. Further adding onto chamomile benefits, the herb is a wonderful for soothing an upset stomach. Helping to soothe and relax the muscles and lining of the intestines, chamomile can help with poor digestion and even those suffering from irritable bowel syndrome (IBS). Promotes Sleep. Drinking chamomile tea soothes the nervous system so is sleep better. It has been used as a solution for insomnia for centuries.

Chaparral Root

An herb derived from the common desert shrubs. Native to the Southwestern United States, Native American healers have for centuries used the leaves and stem of these desert plants. Twentieth century herbalists had come to view chaparral as an effective blood purifier. Has strong anti-inflammation effects and can be applied as an antiseptic to wounds.

Chaste berry (Also known as Vitex) (balances hormones)

An old and trusted "woman's herb" great for easing the discomforts of menstruation and premenstrual syndrome (PMS), including water retention, mood swings, pain, and nervous tension. Flavonoids present in chaste tree are known to slightly increase women's progesterone production, an often lack the cause of menstrual complaints, infertility, heavy bleeding, excessive periods, irregular periods, and no periods. It plays a significant role in hormone regulation, acting directly on the brain's pituitary gland. Menopausal women rely on it as well for alleviating their hormone-related discomforts. *Due to its direct involvement in these hormonal processes, chaste tree is not recommended for use by pregnant women.*

Cinnamon bark

Look for medicinal quality cinnamon, known as Rou Gui, in either Chinese herbal pharmacies or health foods stores. Its pungent sweetness makes it the ideal warming ("yang") tonic for relieving menstrual cramps. Women who find they are chronically cold ("yin"), dry or frail and who may routinely be afflicted with osteoarthritis, asthma or digestive problems will enjoy the greatest benefits from this herbal remedy. *Though its side effects are few, be sure to use cinnamon with caution during pregnancy.*

Cramp Bark

It has been used to relieve cramps of all kinds, including menstrual pains. Relaxes muscles and eases spasms of the lower back and legs. Cramp bark is also said to support uterine function, help regulate excessive blood flow during menstruation and menopause. Helps ease postpartum, uterine, and ovarian pain.

In Hong Kong, an Indonesian maid added her menstrual blood to her employer's food in an attempt to improve their relationship.

Cranberry (Vaccinium macrocarpon)
Best for prevention of Urinary Tract Infections (UTIs)

For reasons that are not well understood, women are more likely than men to develop a urinary tract infection (UTI). In fact, one in five women will get one in her lifetime, according to the National Institute of Diabetes and Digestive and Kidney Diseases. Some women are more prone to UTIs than others — diaphragm users, for instance, are at a substantial risk — and almost 20 percent of women who develop one will eventually develop another. Most infections arise from an overgrowth of E. coli bacteria in the urethra (urethritis) and/or bladder (cystitis). Cranberry prevents bacteria from adhering to the walls of either organ, making it difficult for infection to take hold. It will not, however, kill the bacteria once they are established; in that case, only prescription antibiotics can provide relief.

Damiana
An ancient tonic that lifts the spirits perks up lost vitality and energy and promotes an overall feeling of well-being. It also has a reputation as a sexual stimulant and rejuvenator and has been used to treat sexual impotence and infertility in both males and females. Women have found it helpful when looking for relief of the discomforts of painful menstruation.

Dandelion
Helps eliminate excess water weight associated with PMS and relieves that uncomfortable balloon feeling. Due to its detoxifying effects on the liver, Dandelion can help treat the root cause of the bloating rather than just masking symptoms.

Nearly 15% of menstruating women suffer from debilitating cramps. Scientists claim they have created a pill known as VA 111913 that eliminates most menstrual cramps.

Dong Quai

Or "Female Ginseng," as it is sometimes called is an age-old, natural way to support a woman's health and reproductive system. It is thought to relieve the discomforts of menopause and premenstrual syndrome (PMS) and is useful in addressing irregular cycles and cramping. Dong quai has been used to regulate monthly cycles in women. Naturally high in vitamin B-12, Dong quai contains ferulic acid, a muscle relaxer and pain reliever, as well as blood-thinning chemicals known as coumarins, which work to improve circulation and ensure blood flow to female reproductive organs. Dong quai should be avoided by pregnant women and those suffering from either diarrhea or endometriosis.

Evening Primrose

Contains a high concentration of a fatty acid called GLA. This is essential for cell structure and improved skin elasticity. Has a long tradition of relieving menstrual complaints (including cyclical breast pain) and promotes overall good health?

False Unicorn

Its greatest value came in relieving female disorders of the reproductive organs, including menstrual and menopausal symptoms. It is also thought to help genitourinary complaints and infertility.

Fenugreek (balances hormones)

Is considered the finest herb for enhancing feminine beauty. It also aids in sexual stimulation, balances blood sugar levels, and contains choline which aids in the thinking process. It is particularly useful in the treatment of diabetes and the prevention of breast cancer. Its ability to balance hormone levels helps control the symptoms associated with both PMS and menopause. Fenugreek has been found to promote the growth of new breast cells and increase the size and fullness of the breasts. In addition, the antioxidants contained within Fenugreek help slow the ageing process.

To treat extremely heavy periods, some women turn to uterine ablation [surgical removal of body tissue]. During a uterine ablation, a physician can use several types of methods— such as a laser, a balloon filled with a heated saline solution, electricity, freezing, or microwave—to permanently destroy the endometrium.

Feverfew (Tanacetum parthenium)

Best for Migraines. Three times as many women as men experience migraines, according to the National Headache Foundation. Feverfew may help relieve the nausea and vomiting associated with these debilitating headaches and/ or reduces the need for traditional prophylactic pharmaceuticals, according to Mark Blumenthal, executive director of the American Botanical Council in Austin, Texas. The active agent in feverfew is parthenolide, which may lessen the frequency of headaches in migraine sufferers by reducing inflammation and inhibiting vasoconstriction, according to the NIH; however, more research is needed.

Fo-Ti Root

A soothing, tonic herb that has been used for centuries in China to rejuvenate the body, combat premature aging, and promote longevity. The herb is said to strengthen the liver, kidney, and reproductive systems. Traditional herbalists say it restores vitality, energy, and fertility.

Ginger

This herb is believed to lessen the severity of nausea and vomiting resulting from motion sickness, morning sickness and chemotherapy and it may also decrease joint pain from arthritis. It promotes the release of bile from the gallbladder as well. This herb is recognized by the FDA as being "generally safe." Ginger has blood thinning and cholesterol lowering properties, a characteristic that may help in treating heart disease.

Gotu Kola

Also known as centella and Asiatic, this herb has a reputation for alleviating fatigue and depression, treating memory loss and anxiety.

In America, eight out of ten teen dads don't marry the mother of the child.

Guduchi

Works as a rasayana and promotes the reversal of aging. It is an anti-inflammatory, anti-pyretic and diuretic alterative. Guduchi is used in the treatment of urinary disorders, general debility, autoimmune diseases, and dyspepsia. It also acts as a mild cleanser.

Horse Chestnut

Used to improve the circulatory system. It strengthens capillary walls and dilates blood vessels, which helps to relieve varicose veins, phlebitis, swollen ankles, and local edema. The herb may reduce blood clots and hardening of the arteries.

Horsetail

A healing herb, rich in nutrients and high in silica, which helps the body absorb calcium. It promotes strong, healthy nails, teeth, hair, skin and, most importantly, strong bones. This is particularly beneficial for countering the bone loss and osteoporosis experienced by menopausal women.

Irish Moss

Soothes mucous membranes and alleviates respiratory ailments, such as bronchitis, dry cough, and other lung problems. Like many other bountiful nutrients from the ocean, Irish moss is a wonderful tonic for maintaining youthful, unblemished skin. It has anti-inflammatory effects.

Juniper Berry

Promotes urine flow, helps to clear the kidneys, bladder, and prostate of toxic wastes, while at the same time helping to combat urinary infections in both men and women. Well-known in the kitchen and as a flavoring for gin, juniper berry's warm, aromatic qualities aid digestion. It also helps to relieve arthritis and painful joints.

Kacip Fatimah

Kacip Fatimah is reported to help establish a regular menstrual cycle when periods fail to appear for reasons like stress, illness or when the pill is discontinued. Prevents cramping, water retention and irritability usually associated with PMS. Balances, builds, and harmonizes the female reproductive system to encourage healthy conception. Supports healthy vaginal flora to prevent irritation and infections. Alleviates fatigue, smooths menopausal symptoms, and promote emotional well-being.

Helps establish regular bowel movements (so it may help to clear up your skin) Anti-flatulence, drive away and prevent the formation of gas. Firming and toning of abdominal muscles. Traditionally, Kacip Fatimah is used for enhancing vitality, overcome tiredness and help to tone vaginal muscles for women.

Korean Ginseng

Women have used this to alleviate unpleasant symptoms of menopause. Long considered it to be an overall body tonic, Korean ginseng is believed to vitalize, strengthen, and rejuvenate the entire body.

Lady's Mantle

Lady's Mantle is an astringent herb that works well on hollow organs like the uterus. Rather than toning the uterus, though, Lady's Mantle works to draw out excess fluid and soothe inflammation. *For that reason, this herb is well-suited for consumption after childbirth, during your menstrual cycle and during the delightful time of menopause.* Lady's Mantle's effects are not isolated to the uterus. It works well for mild cases of diarrhea to draw out excess fluid and soothe inflamed intestinal walls (combine it with red raspberry leaf for added relief).

Lavender

Soothe headaches, calm nerves, and stress. Lavender is an antibacterial property for the skin. Moreover, it is an effective tonic that can improve sleep.

Lemon Balm (Melissa)

The herb has been used for centuries to soothe tension. Will not only alleviate stress and anxiety, but is said to improve memory and mental function. It also helps to relieve indigestion.

Licorice

Contains estrogenic compounds and is useful in the treatment of depression. Licorice also reduces stress levels by preventing the breakdown of adrenal hormones such as cortisol, the body's main stress-fighting hormone, making them more available to the body.

Less than two percent of teen moms earn a college degree by age 30.

Lobelia

Recent experiments have claimed that the herb may be helpful to smokers who wish to "quit the habit" and have tried all other remedies without success. It is believed to make the taste of nicotine repulsive. Lobelia may calm the nerves and relax the muscles of the body.

Lodhra

Is astringent, cold, anti-inflammatory and Grahi in properties. It is used in the treatment of diarrhea, dysentery, bleeding piles, hemorrhagea, metrorrhagea, leucorrhea, blood disorders, skin disorders and other uterine disorders. Lodhra is also used to treat skin conditions such as acne, redness, and inflammation.

Maca Root (balances hormones)

Maca is a nourishing food for the endocrine system, aiding both the pituitary, adrenal, and thyroid glands (all involved in hormonal balance.) Maca helps to stimulate and nourish the pituitary gland, acting as a tonic for the hormone system. When the pituitary gland functions optimally, the entire endocrine system becomes balanced, because the pituitary gland controls the hormone output of the other three glands. Maca is a wonderful super food to support overall hormonal balance by providing support and nourishment for the systems that control hormone release and production. It is also used to relieve the symptoms of menopause and premenstrual syndrome (PMS), as well as enhance energy and strength during athletic performance. Used for centuries to increase vitality, promotes libido, fertility and sexual performance and stamina.

Marshmallow Root

Aids the body expel excess fluid. It sooths the mucous membranes. The herb is good for easing bladder infection, digestive upsets, intestinal disorders, kidney problems and sinusitis.

Nineteen out of 100 girls in developing countries gave birth by age 18 and three out of 100 gave birth before age 15.

Mistletoe

The mistletoe leaves and young twigs are used by herbalists for treating circulatory and respiratory problems.

Motherwort

Provides support for women's health, easing menstrual cramps, PMS, and the symptoms of menopause. May help to alleviate stress, depression, anxiety, and nervous disorders as it is also considered a relaxant.

Mullein

Mullein has anti-spasmodic properties that help with menstrual cramps or stomach cramps associated with gastric distress. The anti-inflammatory effects of mullein can help to ease the pain associated with joint or muscle pain by reducing inflammation and swelling. Mullein is a natural anti-inflammatory thanks to the verbascoses it contains. Drinking mullein has been found to help a number of digestive problems including diarrhea, constipation, hemorrhoids, and bladder infections. It is also sometimes used to get rid of intestinal worms. Mullein has natural sedative benefits and may be helpful in the treatment of insomnia and anxiety.

Musta

Is used to treat menstrual disorders such as dysmenorrhea, PMS, irritability, menstrual pain, and the retention of water. It also helps in the treatment of yeast and Candida formation, parasites, sluggish liver, indigestion, dysentery, loss of appetite, chronic fevers, gastrointestinal problems, and menopausal symptoms. Musta also helps to reduce inflammation and heals the skin, making it great for treating breakouts and acne during adolescence.

Myrrh

Known as a powerful natural antiseptic, antibacterial, antiviral, anti-inflammatory and an antifungal. Myrrh has been used to relieve pain and alleviate skin disorders.

During the nineteenth century, it was widely thought that intercourse with a menstruating woman would transmit gonorrhea, which may have been mistaken for trichomoniasis [sexually transmitted disease (STD)]. Trichomoniasis becomes worse during menstruation because of lower vaginal acidity.

Nettle Leaf

Nettle's anti-inflammatory effects have been repeatedly confirmed by modern research. It is particularly effective in treating allergic rhinitis and relieving nearly all the symptoms of itchy, watery eyes, sneezing and runny nose. Has been shown to be a diuretic.

Pennyroyal

Removes gas from the digestive system. Can be used for upset stomachs and may cleanse toxins from the body through the skin. The herb is also used for digestive issues that relieve indigestion, flatulence and grumbling in the intestines. Use only as directed.

Peony Root

Used in herbal medicine for thousands of years for its tranquilizing effect on the nerves, pain relieving effect on muscles and purifying effect on the blood. Best known for its antispasmodic capabilities.

Red Clover Flower (balances hormones)

Called one of "God's greatest blessings to man" and is said to be a wonderful blood purifier and cleanser and has been used to treat serious invasive disease, debilitating wasting diseases, excess mucus in the lungs and elsewhere, irritable bowel, gout, kidney and liver ailments. Helps promote fertility and aids in the treatment of hormonal imbalances, PMS, ovulation, lack of menstruation and painful menstruation. Women who are trying to conceive can utilize red clover for its alkalinizing effects, as it balances vaginal pH in favor of conception.

Red Raspberry Leaf

It is rich in minerals and vitamins that promote the health of hair, skin, nails, bones, and teeth and is said to provide relief for heavy cramping and excessive bleeding during menstruation. Also, useful for PMS symptoms.

Almost 50 percent of teens have never considered how a pregnancy would affect their lives.

Rehmannia Root
Long used in China to replenish vitality, Rehmannia root is becoming popular in the West for fatigue to help with circulation and regulate menstruation.

Sarsaparilla
Has long been used as a blood purifier and tonic that boosts stamina and energy. Sarsaparilla is considered an antibacterial and anti-inflammatory and has a good tonic effect on the body.

Saw Palmetto
Is nourishing to the entire endocrine system. It normalizes reproductive function, is anti-inflammatory and urinary antiseptic. It supports stress and immune system response to treat chronic fatigue.

Shatavari (balances hormones)
Is an asparagus root that is used as a rejuvenative tonic, nutritive, diuretic, antispasmodic, emmenagogue and antacid? Shatavari is considered to be the best herb for the female reproductive system. It is useful for treating infertility, decreased libido, miscarriage, menopause, leucorrhea, dryness in the vaginal wall, and has the ability to balance pH in the cervical area. It contains saponins or phytoestrogens, which has an effect on the female mammary gland.

Siberian Ginseng
It helps to support the body's resistance to infection during prolonged periods of physical and mental stress. Athletes who want to increase performance and endurance favor its stamina-building benefits. Siberian ginseng's stress-fighting capacities have been useful in treating problems with concentration and environmental sensitivity.

Shepherd's Purse
Shepherd's Purse can help regulate blood flow and is often used as an herbal remedy to treat regular bleeding disorders, such as heavy periods. It is used to stop heavy bleeding and hemorrhaging, particularly from the uterus. When taken internally, shepherd's purse can reduce heavy menstrual periods, and it has been used to treat postpartum hemorrhage.

Still, it is considered most effective for the treatment of chronic uterine bleeding disorders, including uterine bleeding due to the presence of a fibroid tumor. Shepherd's purse has also been used internally to treat cases of blood in the urine and bleeding from the gastrointestinal tract, such as with bleeding ulcers. An astringent agent, shepherd's purse constricts blood vessels, thereby reducing blood flow. Shepherd's purse is also thought to cause the uterine muscle to contract, which also helps reduce bleeding.

Skull Cap
A natural way to ease frayed nerves, relax, and get a restful sleep. May help with premenstrual syndrome and monthly cramps. Skull cap is also considered extremely useful for alleviating the difficulties of barbiturate and drug withdrawal.

Slippery Elm Bark
This lubricating and nutritious herb coats irritated areas, allowing the body to heal itself. Its elevated level of mucilage helps to soothe a sore throat, ease indigestion, and lubricate the bowel.

Squaw Vine (balances hormones)
Squaw vine is used for female hormone balance, mild mood changes, cramps, and edema associated with the menstrual cycle, menopause and hot flashes and PMS. It is used to relieve painful menstruation cramps.

Turmeric
Turmeric is one of the most potent natural anti-inflammatories available. Turmeric is used to treat a variety of symptoms associated with menstruation. As a blood mover it moves stagnant blood and reduces clots. It also works as an antispasmodic on smooth muscle tissue, helping to relieve pain associated with cramping.

Uva Ursi
Used for centuries as a mild diuretic with powerful antiseptic qualities that help to remedy a full range of urinary tract infections, such as prostatitis, cystitis, and urethritis It helps to eliminate wastes and toxins.

A study recently released by the National Campaign to Prevent Teen and Unplanned Pregnancy showed that the birth rate of girls in rural counties in 2010—the latest available data—was almost 33% higher than in the rest of the country.

Vitex (Also known as Chaste Berry) (balances hormones)

Vitex supports hormonal balance in the body by having an effect on the hypothalamic-pituitary-ovarian axis (hormonal feedback loop), correcting the problem at the source. Vitex has been found to help normalize ovulation and progesterone levels.

White Willow Bark

Ingredients in white willow bark contain compounds from which aspirin was derived. This natural painkiller contains the beneficial effects of aspirin without the side effects typically associated with synthetic aspirin products.

Wild Yam (balances hormones)

High in plant hormones, which may be synthesized by the body to support its own hormone health. For women who want to continue the normal balance of hormones, benefit from relief of pains and aches or simply enjoy overall good health.

Yarrow

Lab tests show that yarrow contains flavonoids (plant-based chemicals) that increase saliva and stomach acid, helping to improve digestion. Yarrow may also relax smooth muscle in the intestine and uterus, which can relieve stomach and menstrual cramps.

Yerba Maté

Excellent source of vitamins, minerals, and fatty acids. Similar to green tea yet higher in nutritional value. Yerba maté contains 27% more active nutritional compounds than green tea. This is a powerful antioxidant found to stimulate the immune system and aid in protecting against disease."

WHAT ARE DIGESTIVE ENZYMES?

According to Dr. Amy Myers, when you eat, your body has to break down the food into micro and macro nutrients that can then be absorbed and used by your body. Digestive enzymes are small proteins that act on specific molecules within foods to break them down. Most people are familiar with the enzyme lactase, which is responsible for breaking down the milk sugar called lactose. People who are missing this enzyme are not able to digest milk (known as "lactose-intolerance"). Similarly, there are many other enzymes that each work on a specific type of molecule. If you are deficient in any one of these, your body may not be breaking down food as well as it should, which can cause significant issues in the digestive tract.

The digestion process begins in your mouth, where saliva starts breaking down your food. From there your food travels to your stomach, where stomach acid, primarily hydrochloric acid (HCL), begins breaking down proteins. Finally, the majority of digestive enzymes are made by the pancreas. When you eat, the pancreas receives a hormonal signal to release pancreatic juice into the small intestine. Pancreatic juice contains several digestive enzymes, as well as bicarbonate to neutralize the acid from your stomach. The enzymes work in the small intestine to break down the food so it can be absorbed. Enzymes produced by the pancreas include:

- **Amylases** – these break down starches (complex carbohydrates)
- **Lipases** – these break down fats.
- **Proteases and Peptidases** – these break down proteins.

In addition, there are a number of enzymes located near the lining of the small intestine (the brush border), most of which break down disaccharides into simple sugars, which can then be absorbed from the intestines into the bloodstream.

How Do Digestive Enzymes Affect Gut Health?

As said by some Dr. Amy Myers, M.D., you are not what you eat, you are what you digest and absorb. If your food is not properly digested and absorbed in your small intestines, this can lead to malnourishment, because not enough nutrients are being absorbed by your body. In addition, the undigested food travels down through the digestive tract and provides food for the "bad" bacteria, causing gas and bloating, and leading to **dysbiosis** as the bad bacteria thrive and outnumber the good bacteria. The amount and type of undigested food that reaches the large intestine may have an important impact on the balance of good and bad bacteria in the colon.

What Causes Digestive Enzyme Deficiency?

Now that we understand the importance of digestive enzymes, let us look at what causes digestive enzyme deficiency. Conventional medicine only recognizes a few causes of digestive enzyme deficiency, and they are only the most extreme cases, including acute or chronic pancreatitis, cystic fibrosis, cancer of the pancreas, gallbladder removal, and diseases of the small intestine that affect the brush border, such as Crohn's or celiac disease. Functional medicine, on the other hand, recognizes that there are many underlying health issues that can contribute to enzyme deficiency. **Leaky gut** is the most common culprit, since it destroys the brush border of your small intestines. Inflammation from food sensitivities and toxins also decreases enzyme production, as well as **chronic stress**, genetics, and aging. Low stomach acid also plays a role because an acidic environment is necessary to activate the enzymes responsible for protein digestion.

Beyond the wider scope of causes, functional medicine also differs from conventional medicine in that conventional medicine views enzyme deficiency as a black and white issue, you have "normal" levels, or you are severely deficient. In functional medicine, we see wellness as a spectrum, and recognize that just because you are not to the point of severe deficiency, doesn't mean that your levels are optimal or that your health won't improve by increasing them.

In my experience as a physician, I have found that increasing digestive enzymes eases the burden of many of the most common root causes of chronic disease, including leaky gut, infections such as **Candida** or SIBO (Small Intestine Bacterial Overgrowth), and chronic inflammation caused by a poor diet.

How Do You Treat Digestive Enzyme Deficiency?

In functional medicine, we use the 4R Approach to heal your gut, and replenishing your digestive enzymes through a **digestive enzyme supplement** is a key part of step number two, restore the good. Restoring digestive enzymes not only ensures that you properly break down and absorb the nutrients from your food, a recent study showed that digestive enzymes may improve not only gastrointestinal symptoms, but also behavioral symptoms in children with autism.

So, if you are overcoming a leaky gut, transitioning from a diet of processed foods, having digestive issues such as gas, bloating, indigestion, reflux, diarrhea, constipation, or undigested food in your stool, digestive enzymes are recommended. Choose a supplement that contains a complete range of enzymes, such as my Complete Enzymes formula, which is also available in a chewable form.

Should You Be Taking Digestive Enzymes?

Are you trying to repair a leaky gut? Do you suffer from chronic digestive issues such as gas, bloating, indigestion, or constipation? Do you experience reflux after a meal? Or do you see pieces of undigested food or a fatty substance in your stool? If so, your body may not be producing enough digestive enzymes, or your enzymes may not be working as well as they should.

PREBIOTICS VS. PROBIOTICS

Prebiotics are not *Probiotics.*

"While the general public has long understood probiotics, prebiotics are less known. But there are significant differences between the two, including health benefits. Probiotics are live bacteria in yogurt, other dairy products, and pills. Doctors often prescribe probiotics to patients on antibiotics in an attempt to combat gastrointestinal side effects of the medication. And while probiotics have been shown effective in managing certain gastrointestinal conditions, they do not have the same power that prebiotics do.

First, they're delicate — heat and stomach acid can kill them, rendering them ineffective before they've even been digested. Also, those who do not eat dairy foods for taste or dietary reasons may find ingesting adequate amounts of probiotics difficult, if not impossible. Finally, we do not know which "good" bacteria our unique bodies would benefit from. For some people, a certain good bacterial strain would be helpful. For others, it may not. When we consume probiotics, we are taking a guess at which bacteria might be helpful and hoping for the best. We are also hoping the ones that make it past the heat and acid of our stomach will actually go on to provide some health benefits to our system.

If this is a probiotic then what is a prebiotic? In short, the prebiotic is a specialized plant fiber that beneficially nourishes the good bacteria already in the large bowel or colon. While probiotics introduce beneficial bacteria into the gut, prebiotics function as a fertilizer for the beneficial bacteria that is already there. They help your healthy bacteria grow, improving the good to-bad bacteria ratio. This ratio has been shown to have a direct correlation to your health and overall wellbeing, from your stomach to your brain.

The body itself does not digest these plant fibers. Instead, it uses these fibers to promote the growth of many of the healthy bacteria in the gut. These, in turn, provide many digestive and general health benefits. Recent studies have also shown prebiotics and good bacterial gut balance play a direct role in mental health. Individuals who consume prebiotics on a daily basis have fewer issues with anxiety, depression, and stress. In fact, when their saliva was evaluated, it contained lower levels of cortisol. Prominent levels of this hormone have been linked directly to mental health disorders.

Prebiotics, unlike probiotics, are not destroyed in the body. Heat or bacteria do not affect them. Getting the full benefits of prebiotics is easy, especially when consumed in a full-spectrum supplement form."

Probiotic vs Prebiotic

According to Dr. Frank Jackson of Prebiotin Academy, prebiotics and probiotics both accomplish important health tasks for the human gut. Trying to decide between a probiotic and prebiotic supplement regimen? Consider these prebiotics vs probiotics facts:

PREBIOTIC VS PROBIOTIC

PREBIOTICS

PREBIOTICS are a special form of dietary fiber that acts as a fertilizer for the healthy bacteria in your gut.

PREBIOTIC powders are not affected by heat, cold, acid or time.

PREBIOTICS provide a wide range of health benefits to the otherwise healthy person. Most of these have been medically proven.

PREBIOTICS nourish the healthy bacteria that everyone already has in their gut.

PROBIOTICS

PROBIOTICS are live bacteria in yogurt, dairy products, and pills. There are hundreds of probiotic species available. Which of the hundreds of available probiotics is best for the average healthy person is still unknown?

PROBIOTIC bacteria must be kept alive. They may be killed by heat, stomach acid or simply die with time.

PROBIOTICS are still not clearly known to provide health benefits to the otherwise healthy. Some are suspected but still not proven.

PROBIOTICS must compete with the over 1000 bacteria species already in the gut.

PREBIOTICS may be helpful for several chronic digestive disorders or inflammatory bowel disease.

Certain PROBIOTIC species have been shown to be helpful for childhood diarrhea, irritable bowel disease and for recurrence of certain bowel infections such as C. difficile.

Science has proven the health benefits of prebiotics include increased bone density, strengthened immune system, better-controlled weight and appetite, and improved bowel regularity. **Recent studies** have also found that individuals taking prebiotics experience improved mental health.

Consuming Prebiotic Fiber

Chicory Root has the highest percentage of Prebiotic Fiber per gram. Live probiotic bacteria are easy to find and consume if dairy products are to your taste and meet your dietary needs. Yogurt, for example, contains probiotics; but where can you find prebiotic fiber? It is easy if you know where to look.

Prebiotic fiber is found in many fruits and vegetables, such as the skin of apples, bananas, onions and garlic, Jerusalem artichoke, chicory root, and beans. Sounds easy to get enough prebiotic fiber, right? Unfortunately, the minute amounts of fiber in each of these foods — such as 1 to 2 grams per serving — make ingesting enough fiber extremely difficult. Most people should consume at least 25 grams of fiber every day, and the foods highest in prebiotic fiber — chicory root is one such example — are nearly impossible to eat in large quantities every day. The good news is that adding a prebiotic fiber supplement to your diet is fast and simple. In supplement form, prebiotic fiber is also mild in texture and tasteless, making it easy to add to water, cereal or any other food. Simply sprinkle it on your foods or in your favorite drinks to enjoy the many benefits. Prebiotin makes it even easier — you can buy it in on-the-go, single-serving packets that are perfect for a busy lifestyle.

How Prebiotics Help

For years, hardly anyone in the medical profession paid any attention to the role the colon plays in overall health. Over the past 15 years, however, we have discovered that the colon — and specifically, the bacteria that call the colon home — is incredibly important to wellness. The healthy bacteria that live there strengthen the bowel wall, improve mineral absorption and aid in the regulation of hormone production, which has a range of essential benefits. Prebiotics fertilize these beneficial bacteria as they stifle production of the bad, disease-causing bacteria, and Prebiotin prebiotic fiber is independently shown to cause the multiplication of beneficial bacteria which combat gut dysbiosis.

> **(Dysbiosis (dis·bē·ō⍰·sis),** *n* an imbalance in the intestinal bacteria that precipitates changes in the normal activities of the gastrointestinal tractor vagina, possibly resulting in health problems.

> Also called *dyssymbiosis*. The condition that results when the natural flora of the gut is thrown out of balance, such as when antibiotics are taken.

When you have ample beneficial bacteria, you can experience better overall health from a physical, mental and emotional standpoint. You will be better nourished, feel fuller, and able to achieve and maintain a healthy weight more easily.

Can You Take Probiotics and Prebiotics Together?

Yes, you can take probiotics and prebiotics together. Prebiotics do not negatively interact with probiotics. Prebiotics do not interfere with medications, either. High-quality probiotics and prebiotics are safe when taken together.

In fact, when you think about how probiotics and prebiotics work, it makes sense to take them together. Simply put, prebiotics are "food" for probiotics. Probiotics digest prebiotics and use the molecules as energy. In some ways, probiotics and prebiotics act *synergistically* for gut health.

When Is the Best Time to Take Prebiotics and Probiotics?

The best time to take prebiotics and probiotics is regularly. Follow the recommendations for each one, take them at the same time each day and take them consistently. Some sources have suggested that prebiotics should be taken before probiotics. The truth is that it really does not matter.

The body "processes" prebiotics and probiotics at different rates. It may take hours for prebiotics and probiotics to make their way to the large intestine. They may not travel through the intestines at the same rate. In fact, most probiotics die in the stomach acid and never make it to the large intestine at all. So, trying to precisely schedule the best time to take prebiotics and probiotics together is rather pointless. The good news is that there are bacteria in the large intestine ready to digest the prebiotics once they arrive.

When Is the Best Time to Take Prebiotics?

Again, consistency is the key to taking prebiotics. You want to provide the healthy microbes in your digestive tract with a steady supply of "food." Just as you like to eat at the same time each day, healthy gut bacteria come to expect a consistent supply of nutrients. If you starve the bacteria, they will either stop multiplying or die off, opening the door to unhealthy bacteria. Make a schedule to take prebiotics, and then stick with it.

Many people find that prebiotics make them feel fuller, faster. In fact, this satiety has been shown in **research studies and clinical trials**. Therefore, people who are trying to maintain a healthy weight or lose weight could take prebiotics along with meals. Prebiotics can help people feel full even if they have eaten less.

When Is the Best Time to Take Probiotics?

Probiotics are mostly destroyed by stomach acid and digestive enzymes. People can help protect against this destruction by taking probiotics with meals. The food may function as a buffer to protect the probiotics as they make their way through the stomach and small intestine. On the other hand, digestion is increased during and immediately after a meal. Thus, eating could make a more hostile environment for the probiotics. One way to overcome each of these problems is to take enough active probiotic colonies so that at least some of them make it to the large intestine.

Prebiotics vs. Probiotics: Which Is Better?

Both prebiotics and probiotics can benefit human health. However, probiotics suffer from one major problem: they have a challenging time making it from the mouth to the large intestine. Compared to what was swallowed, only a small number of living probiotic organisms reaches the gut.

Prebiotics, on the other hand, are not digested by the human body, but are instead digested by gut bacteria. For prebiotics, what you eat is what you get. Prebiotics support the growth of healthy bacteria already in the large intestine. In some ways, probiotics are unnecessary for healthy individuals who consistently take prebiotics. For these reasons, prebiotics are better than probiotics for most people.

PREGNANCY

"Now that you have a basic understanding of the reproductive system and its nutritional needs for optimal health, what if you become pregnant? Again, as defined in the vocabulary, pregnancy is the process of human gestation that takes place in the female's body as a fetus develops, from fertilization to birth (*see* parturition). It begins when a viable sperm from the male and egg from the ovary merge in the fallopian tube (*see* fertilized). The fertilized egg (zygote) grows by cell division as it moves toward the uterus, where it implants in the lining and grows into an embryo and then a fetus. A placenta and umbilical cord develop for nutrient and waste exchange between the circulations of mother and fetus. A protective fluid-filled amniotic sac encloses and cushions the fetus.

Missed Period
One of the first signs of pregnancy may be that you do not have your monthly period.

Pregnancy Tests
Pregnancy tests look for the human chorionic gonadotropin (hCG) hormone which is also called the pregnancy hormone. Human chorionic gonadotropin (hCG) is a special hormone in the urine or blood that is only there when a woman is pregnant.

1. The pregnancy hormone is made in your body when a fertilized egg implants in the uterus. This usually happens about six days after conception (when the egg is fertilized when having sex). The amount of pregnancy hormone increases with each day that you are pregnant.

2. There are two types of pregnancy tests. One evaluates the blood for the pregnancy hormone, hCG. The other checks the urine for this

hormone. You can do a urine test at home with a home pregnancy test. Most women first use home pregnancy tests to find out if they are pregnant.

3. If a home pregnancy test says you are pregnant or you think you might be pregnant, you should call your health care provider right away! Your health care provider can use a more sensitive test along with an examination to tell for sure if you are pregnant. Seeing your health care provider early in your pregnancy will help you and your baby stay healthy.

THE FIRST TRIMESTER

The first trimester of pregnancy is the time from the start of your pregnancy to 12 weeks. During the first trimester you may experience swollen breasts, tiredness (fatigue), nausea and vomiting (morning sickness), backaches, mood swings and frequent urination. Most pregnant women have monthly prenatal visits with their health care provider until the end of this trimester.

During the first trimester your health care provider will:
*   Check your weight, blood pressure, and urine;
*   Check the size and shape of your uterus;
*   Check your hands and feet for swelling;
*   Toward the end of the first trimester, listen to your baby's heartbeat.

THE SECOND TRIMESTER

The second trimester of pregnancy goes from the 13th week to the 27th week. In the second trimester, there is usually less nausea and tiredness (fatigue) than in the first trimester. The baby grows rapidly and by the end of the second trimester you begin to feel the baby move. As the baby grows, the uterus also grows and rises higher in the abdomen during the second trimester. Some women find that they do not have to urinate as frequently as before. However, you may feel pressure in your abdomen or backaches or shortness of breath. On average, it is normal to gain about one pound per week, or about three to four pounds per month during this trimester. Most pregnant women have monthly prenatal visits with their health care provider until the end of this trimester.

During the second trimester your health care provider will:
- Check your weight, blood pressure, and urine;
- Check the size and shape of your uterus and listen to the baby's heartbeat.
- Check your hands and feet for swelling;
- Check your legs for varicose veins;
- Do other tests to check for any potential problems.

THE THIRD TRIMESTER

This is the last trimester, running from the 28th week until the 40th week when your baby is born. You may feel tired again during the third trimester and many women find breathing more difficult and notice they have to go to the bathroom more often. This is because the baby is getting bigger, and it is putting more pressure on your organs including your lungs and bladder. On average, it is normal to gain about one pound per week, or three to four pounds per month, during the third trimester. By the end of your pregnancy, you should have gained on average, 25 to 30 pounds. From 30 weeks to 38 weeks of pregnancy, most health care providers recommend one office visit every two weeks. After 38 weeks, women normally see their health care provider every week until delivery.

During the third trimester your health care provider will:
- Check your weight, blood pressure, and urine;
- Check the size and shape of your uterus and listen to the baby's heartbeat;
- Check the baby's position;
- Check your hands and feet for swelling and legs for varicose veins;
- Do other tests to check for any foreseeable problems.

Call your health care provider right away if you have any of the following symptoms:
- Warm fluid flows out of your vagina, your "water breaks."
- Bleeding from your vagina.
- Sharp severe pain in your back or abdomen.
- Severe headache, blurred vision, or slurred speech."

Pregnancy Month to Month

BABY'S GROWTH MONTH ONE

Weeks 1 & 2

According to Dr NDTV, the average length of gestation is 266 days, which means your baby will be born around 38 weeks after conception. Because many women are not familiar with their fertility cues and do not know when conception happened, pregnancy is measured from the first day of the last menstrual period. The average length of pregnancy is 280 days, which means your baby will be born around 40 weeks after the first day of your last menstrual period. By this standard of measuring, your first two weeks of pregnancy happen before your child is conceived.

During this time, the egg that will become your child begins the maturation process and the sperm that will become your child is being produced.

Week 3

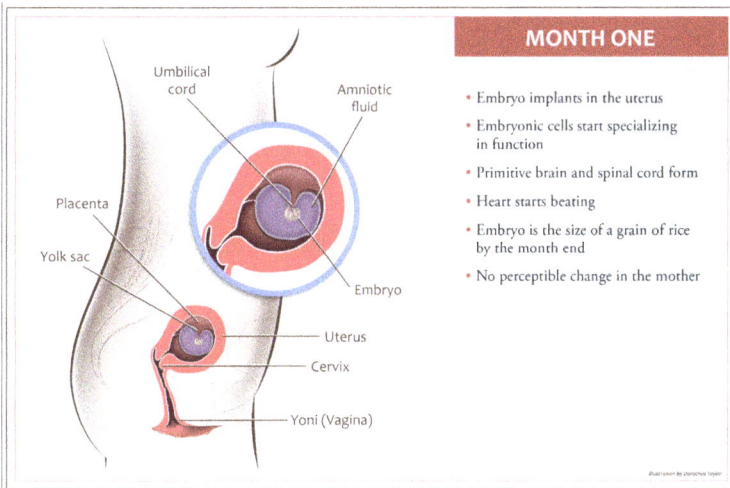

MONTH ONE

- Embryo implants in the uterus
- Embryonic cells start specializing in function
- Primitive brain and spinal cord form
- Heart starts beating
- Embryo is the size of a grain of rice by the month end
- No perceptible change in the mother

This is the week the sperm and egg meet. Some of the decisions about your child, such as gender and if he or she will have any chromosomal problems, will be decided at conception. After the sperm and egg combined, your newly created baby begins a process of cell division that could rightly be called "explosive." In these first weeks, perhaps before you even realize you are pregnant, your baby has begun to develop everything it needs to survive until birth. By the third week of life your baby 's heart is already pumping blood on its own.

Week 4

The creation of your baby begins before he is even attached to your uterine lining. As the egg divides and grows, cells begin to be specialized. The fertilized egg will create your baby, the placenta, the amniotic sac, and the amniotic fluid. Approximately 10 days after fertilization, your baby implants in the uterus. The lungs, heart and spinal cord begin to form. By the end of the fourth week your baby is less than .03 oz, and is approximately 1/8 of an inch long.

BABY'S GROWTH MONTH TWO

Week 5

In this second month of life, your baby continues to develop internal organs and other major structures of the body. There is also continued growth and development of the brain and spinal column. Your baby's heart is developing along with a primitive circulatory system. By the end of this week your baby's heart will begin beating! For the next few weeks, your baby will be at the Embryo stage of development.

Week 6

Your baby has tripled his size this week, measuring ¼ inch (4-6 mm) from head to bottom, also called crown to rump. Babies are not usually measured head to toe before being born because of the difficulty in measuring the curled-up legs. If you could see your baby now you would see arm and leg buds on the sides of the body, eyes forming on the sides of the head and an opening for the mouth being formed.

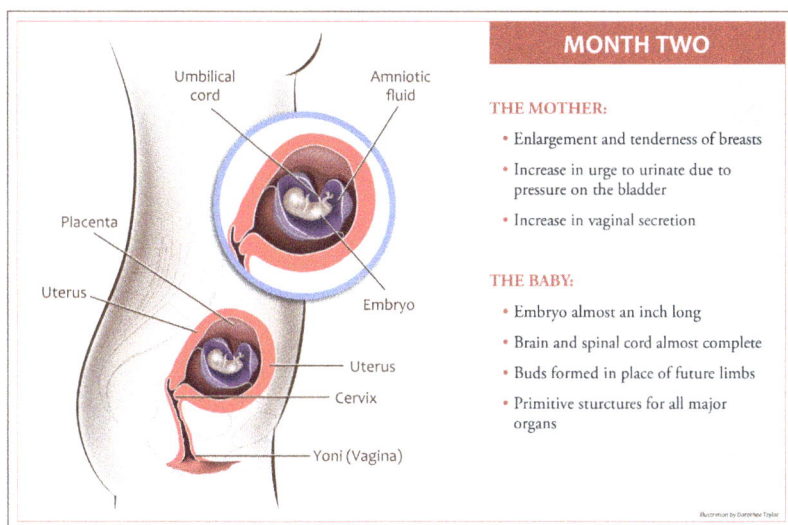

MONTH TWO

Umbilical cord

Amniotic fluid

Placenta

Uterus

Embryo

Uterus

Cervix

Yoni (Vagina)

THE MOTHER:
- Enlargement and tenderness of breasts
- Increase in urge to urinate due to pressure on the bladder
- Increase in vaginal secretion

THE BABY:
- Embryo almost an inch long
- Brain and spinal cord almost complete
- Buds formed in place of future limbs
- Primitive sturctures for all major organs

Illustration by Gutenher Taylor

Week 7

If you could see your baby at this point, you would find the arm and leg buds have lengthened and the arm is divided into a shoulder section and an arm/hand section but there are no fingers yet. Your baby's eyes and nostrils are developing, but the eyes look large and are always open and the nostrils are just nasal pits not a nose yet. His heart bulges out of his chest and the umbilical cord is continuing to lengthen.

Week 8

Internally, your baby is continuing to develop organ systems. Her bronchial tubes (main passages of the lungs) are beginning to branch out and her bones may begin to harden (ossification). Her heart rate is about 150 bpm, which is about twice the speed of an adult heart. She is also developing her pituitary gland, and the gonads are developing into ovaries or testes. By the end of the eighth week, all the organs are present. There is also continued growth and development of the brain and spinal column. At the end of the eighth week your baby will be around 1 inch long and weigh 0.1 oz.

BABY'S GROWTH MONTH THREE

Week 9

Internally, digestive organs are forming. The pancreas, bile ducts and gallbladder have formed by this point. The reproductive organs are also forming, but the external genitalia are not developed yet so you will need to wait to guess the sex by ultrasound.

Week 10

Her upper lip is fully formed, and tooth buds are forming in her gums. She is beginning a time of rapid brain growth, so be sure to continue with good nutrition. If your baby is a boy, his testes are functioning enough to produce testosterone. At this point she is about 1.25 to 1.68 inches (27-35 mm) from crown to rump, and still weighs only .18 oz (5 grams).

Week 11

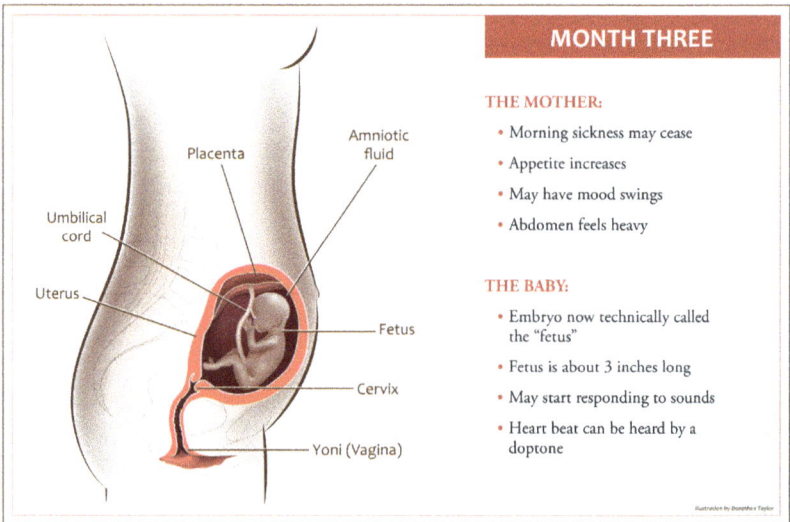

MONTH THREE

THE MOTHER:
- Morning sickness may cease
- Appetite increases
- May have mood swings
- Abdomen feels heavy

THE BABY:
- Embryo now technically called the "fetus"
- Fetus is about 3 inches long
- May start responding to sounds
- Heart beat can be heard by a doptone

Your baby has a definite mini-human look, although the head makes up about half of his total length. He is still completing his development, with fingernails appearing this week. As his eyes mature this week, they develop the iris. The placental blood vessels increase in size to provide more nutrients to your quickly developing baby.

Week 12

By the end of this month your baby will look like a mini human. The face is formed, complete with 32 permanent teeth buds. There are even nails at the end of the fingers and toes. There are also major hormonal changes taking place around this time. Her pituitary gland is mature enough to begin producing hormones, and the placenta is mature enough to take over the production of pregnancy hormones. At the end of the twelfth week your baby will be around 3.5 inches long and weigh 1.7 oz.

Week 13

Your baby's face begins to look more human now, as the face widens to allow the eyes to face the front rather than the sides. He may begin putting his thumb in his mouth as the sucking muscles begin developing. He is also beginning to form skull bones, although these bones are not hardening yet.

BABY'S GROWTH MONTH FOUR

Week 14

Her thyroid gland has matured and is now able to produce hormones. The digestive system is mature enough to produce and eliminate urine into the amniotic fluid. Not only does she drink the amniotic fluid, but practices breathing it too.

Week 15

His eyes and ears are almost in position now. If he will have dark hair, hair follicles may begin to make the pigment. As his hair comes in, a scalp hair pattern is developing. His bones and muscles continue to mature, and he is developing new skills. By now he can make a fist.

Week 16

Your baby is beginning to gain control of her muscle movements. She can even make facial expressions in response to changes in the uterine environment. An experienced mother may be able to begin recognizing the feelings of movement as she exercises her muscles. First time mothers may need to wait a few more weeks before they are certain they are feeling movement. Baby is now big enough that his heartbeat can be heard with a regular stethoscope.

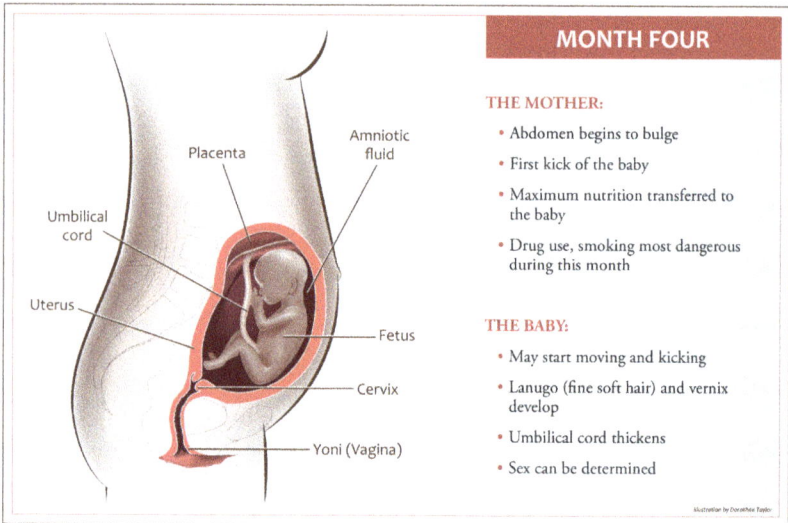

MONTH FOUR

THE MOTHER:
- Abdomen begins to bulge
- First kick of the baby
- Maximum nutrition transferred to the baby
- Drug use, smoking most dangerous during this month

THE BABY:
- May start moving and kicking
- Lanugo (fine soft hair) and vernix develop
- Umbilical cord thickens
- Sex can be determined

Labels: Placenta, Amniotic fluid, Umbilical cord, Uterus, Fetus, Cervix, Yoni (Vagina)

Illustration by Dorothea Taylor

Week 17

The placenta will continue to grow throughout the pregnancy to meet your baby's increasing demands for oxygen, nutrients, and elimination of waste. At this point, the placenta is about 1 (25 mm) inch thick. To help your baby maintain proper body temperature, he is developing a special type of fat called brown fat. It will make up about 2.5% of his weight at birth and will slowly go away after he is born.

BABY'S GROWTH MONTH FIVE

Week 18

Two exciting things happen around this week: your baby may be developed enough to see and to hear. Your baby uses these skills before she is born as a way to familiarize herself with the environment, she will live in. Although her eyes are only able to detect the difference between bright light and darkness, this helps her learn about the day/night schedule where you live.

The sounds she hears are muffled because of the amniotic fluid, but she does hear enough to become familiar with the voice of her mother and others who live in her home. She may also become familiar with the type of music you listen to.

Week 19

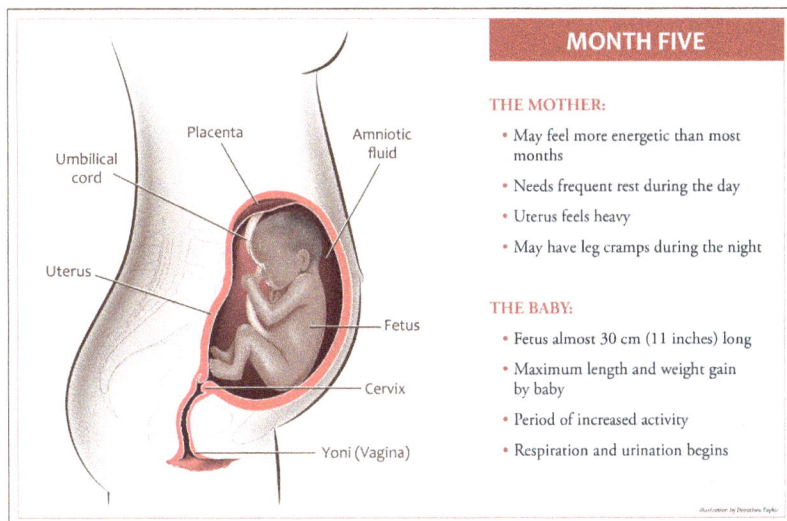

MONTH FIVE

THE MOTHER:
- May feel more energetic than most months
- Needs frequent rest during the day
- Uterus feels heavy
- May have leg cramps during the night

THE BABY:
- Fetus almost 30 cm (11 inches) long
- Maximum length and weight gain by baby
- Period of increased activity
- Respiration and urination begins

Illustration by Denzshia Taylo

Labels: Umbilical cord, Placenta, Amniotic fluid, Uterus, Fetus, Cervix, Yoni (Vagina)

Your baby has been developing two forms of protection for his skin; lanugo hair and vernix caseosa. The vernix is a thick and creamy white substance that prevents the amniotic fluid from damaging the skin. It slowly wears off near the end of your pregnancy, so babies born early tend to have more on their skin than babies born late. Lanugo hair develops all over the body and seems to help the vernix remain attached to the skin. The lanugo will also fall off near the end of your pregnancy.

Week 20

Her skin is developing the layers it needs to provide protection to the bones, muscles, and other tissues underneath. This thickening process will make her skin opaque (you will not be able to see through it any more).At the end of the 20th week your baby will be around 7.5 inches from crown to rump and weigh one pound, and baby's kidneys are now functioning well enough that they can make urine.

Week 21

As the bones are hardening, the bone marrow is also developing. It is now developing the ability to produce blood cells (this is the function of marrow in an adult). Until the marrow can do this on its own, your baby's liver and spleen are making his blood.

BABY'S GROWTH MONTH SIX

Week 22

Your baby is developing two more senses, taste, and touch. All her organ systems are in place, but the specialization and maturation of the systems is continuing. If your baby is a girl, her reproductive organs have formed and are in the proper place. If your baby is a boy, his testes are beginning the descent from the abdomen to their proper place in the scrotum.

Week 23

The bones in your baby's middle ear are hardening, which is necessary for proper hearing and balance. Over the next few weeks, you may find him responding more frequently to the sounds and noises around you.

Week 24

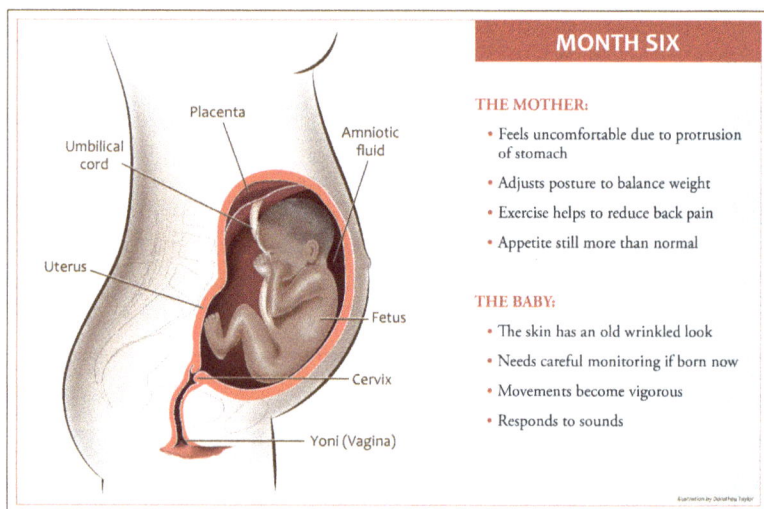

MONTH SIX

Placenta
Amniotic fluid
Umbilical cord
Uterus
Fetus
Cervix
Yoni (Vagina)

THE MOTHER:
- Feels uncomfortable due to protrusion of stomach
- Adjusts posture to balance weight
- Exercise helps to reduce back pain
- Appetite still more than normal

THE BABY:
- The skin has an old wrinkled look
- Needs careful monitoring if born now
- Movements become vigorous
- Responds to sounds

Her lungs are beginning to produce a substance called surfactant. Surfactant is necessary for the lungs to function properly because it prevents the walls of the lungs from sticking to each other when she exhales. The development of the lungs is a lengthy process and will not be complete until she is almost ready to be born. His body has caught up with his head, and although the head is still large compared to an adult, your baby's body and head are in the right proportions for a newborn. At the end of the 24th week your baby will be around 10 inches from crown to rump and weigh 2 pounds.

Week 25

About this time, your baby's spine will begin to form. The spine helps to protect the spinal cord and helps to support your baby in upright positions. The bones and muscles of his hand are developed enough now that he can clench his fingers into a fist.

Week 26

This week her eyes will begin the process of reopening and she will be able to see. Her brain wave patterns for vision and hearing are similar to a newborn at this point.

BABY'S GROWTH MONTH SEVEN

Week 27

Your baby is at a point of rapid brain growth, and he still needs to mature several systems. The lungs and liver are continuing their development, and the immune system is improving.

Week 28

The rapid brain growth that started last week is continuing. Not only is the amount of brain tissue increasing, but the brain design is becoming more mature. It is forming the grooves and indentations characteristic of a human brain.

Week 29

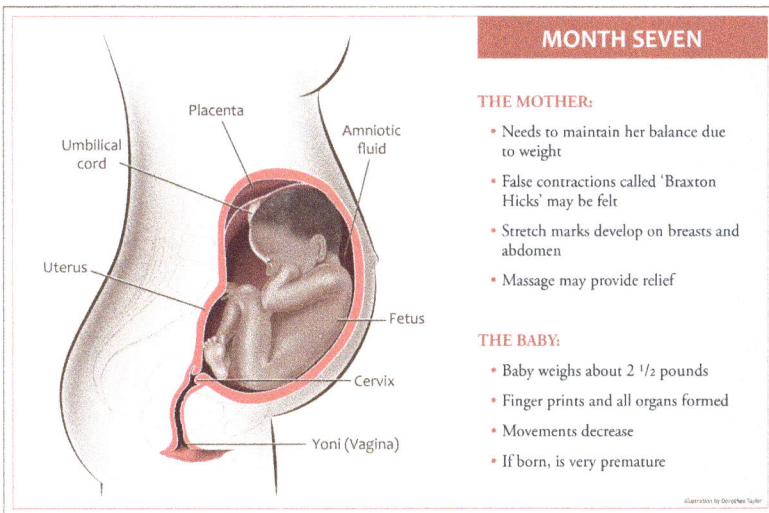

MONTH SEVEN

Placenta
Umbilical cord
Amniotic fluid
Uterus
Fetus
Cervix
Yoni (Vagina)

THE MOTHER:
- Needs to maintain her balance due to weight
- False contractions called 'Braxton Hicks' may be felt
- Stretch marks develop on breasts and abdomen
- Massage may provide relief

THE BABY:
- Baby weighs about 2 1/2 pounds
- Finger prints and all organs formed
- Movements decrease
- If born, is very premature

Illustration by Dorothea Taylor

Your baby will continue to accumulate fat this week which will help to plump him up. If you could look at him, you would notice that his eyes can now move in the sockets – he can look around without turning his head.

Week 30

While she practices working her muscles, her lungs continue to build a supply of surfactant. There is a protein in the surfactant that some experts believe triggers hormonal changes in the mother and baby. These hormonal changes are the beginning stages of your body preparing to give birth. This week your baby is about 3 pounds (1360 grams) and is about 17 inches (38 cm) total length. From head to rump, she is about 11 inches (28 cm). Over the next few weeks, she will continue to gain weight as her body prepares for life outside the womb.

BABY'S GROWTH MONTH EIGHT

Week 31

Over the next two weeks he will mature enough that his chances of survival if born early will be surprisingly good. About 30% of triplets and 10% of twins are born at this time, however most often it is best for babies to stay in the uterus as long as possible.

Week 32

In addition to looking like a newborn, your baby is beginning to react like a newborn. All five of her senses are now functioning. Your baby can see differences of light and dark through your skin, can hear what happens around you and within you, tastes the amniotic fluid, and feels the closeness of your uterine wall. This is also a peak week of movement for your baby. Soon, her size will restrict her to shifting instead of all-out kicks.

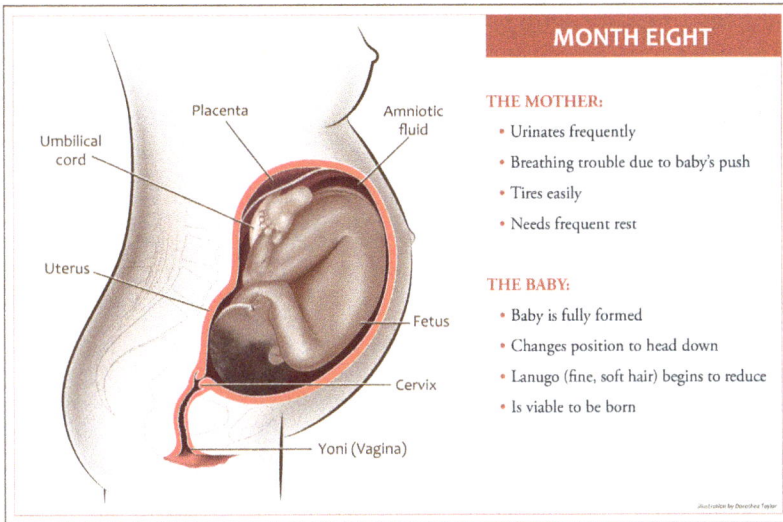

MONTH EIGHT

THE MOTHER:
• Urinates frequently
• Breathing trouble due to baby's push
• Tires easily
• Needs frequent rest

THE BABY:
• Baby is fully formed
• Changes position to head down
• Lanugo (fine, soft hair) begins to reduce
• Is viable to be born

Placenta
Umbilical cord
Amniotic fluid
Uterus
Fetus
Cervix
Yoni (Vagina)

Illustration by Dorothea Taylor

Week 33

Another exciting change in your baby's brain is he now experiences REM (Rapid Eye Movement) sleep. This is the deep stage of sleep where dreaming occurs. He sleeps a lot too. You have probably begun to be familiar with his daily patterns of awake and sleep just by paying attention to his movements.

Week 34

Her body is very mature, and her lungs are well-developed which gives her good chances of survival if she were born this week. The vernix (white substance protecting her skin) is thicker, while the lanugo hair is almost completely gone. Her fingernails have grown to the end of her fingers, and she urinates almost a pint of fluid a day.

Week 35

There is a wide variation in the size of babies by this time. The average is around 5.5 pounds (2550 g) and about 20.25 inches (45 cm) long. You are entering the time of most rapid weight gain, where your baby will be gaining ½ to ¾ of a pound each week. Fat is being deposited all over her body, and the finishing touches are being made to all the organ systems.

BABY'S GROWTH MONTH NINE

Week 36

Your uterus is probably up under your ribs, and you may be feeling that you have run out of room. This is normal, and to be expected since your baby is now about 20.7 inches (46 cm) long and weighs in around six pounds (2750 g). Babies vary in weight from 3 to 6.5 pounds at this point, with the size depending on a number of variables including genetics, the mother's nutrition, and overall health.

Week 37

His lungs are completing the maturation process, and he continues to practice his breathing movements. His muscle and brain development are enough that he can grasp things in his fingers and turn his body towards a source of light.

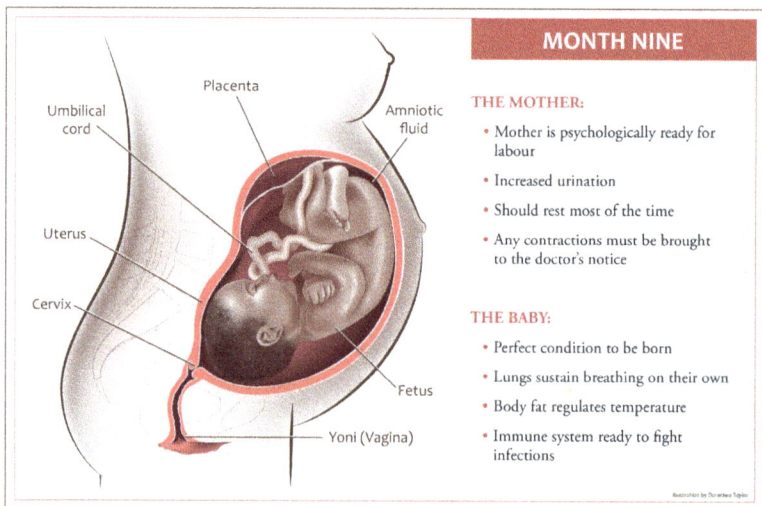

MONTH NINE

Placenta
Umbilical cord
Amniotic fluid
Uterus
Cervix
Fetus
Yoni (Vagina)

THE MOTHER:
- Mother is psychologically ready for labour
- Increased urination
- Should rest most of the time
- Any contractions must be brought to the doctor's notice

THE BABY:
- Perfect condition to be born
- Lungs sustain breathing on their own
- Body fat regulates temperature
- Immune system ready to fight infections

Week 38

If your baby is a boy, his testicles have descended into the scrotum now. If your baby is a girl, her labia have developed. Because she has been practicing sucking and swallowing with the amniotic fluid, there is beginning to be a build-up of waste materials in the intestines. This material is called meconium, and will be your baby's first bowel movements.

Week 39

Your baby is increasing surfactant production for the lungs to prepare for labor. He is also benefiting from your antibodies, which are supplied to him through the placenta. Most of the lanugo hair is gone, and the vernix is disappearing.

Week 40

Your baby is practically ready to be born. A few last details to give him a great start in the world beyond your womb and he is on his way. At the end of the 40th week your baby will be around 14-15 inches from crown to rump and weigh about 6-8 pounds."

About a quarter of teen moms have a second child within 24 months of their first baby.

WILL THE FETUS BE FEMALE OR MALE? WHAT DETERMINES THE SEX?

According to Medical Doctor, Jewel Pookrum (M.D.), male and female development is the same embryologically until the seventh week of pregnancy (gestation). At this time, the presence or absence of the Y chromosome will determine whether the embryo's future development will transform the cells to become male or female. If there is a Y chromosome in the library (nucleus) of the cell, all of the cells of the embryo will commit to becoming male in orientation and function.

The male and female genitalia are the same:

1. The labia majora of the female is the same as the male scrotum or testicular sack.
2. The testicles of the male are the same as the ovaries of the female.
3. The penile shaft in males is the same as the erectile tissue in the female clitoris.
4. The gland's penis also known as the head of the penis is the same as the gland's clitoris.
5. The foreskin of the penis is the same as the prepuce in the females, which is the skin that covers the clitoris.
6. The uterus of the female is the same as the prostate gland of males.

What is a chromosome?

According to NIH National Human Genome Research Institute, chromosomes are thread-like structures located inside the nucleus of animal and plant cells. Each chromosome is made of protein and a single molecule of deoxyribonucleic acid (DNA). Passed from parents to offspring, DNA contains the specific instructions that make each type of living creature unique.

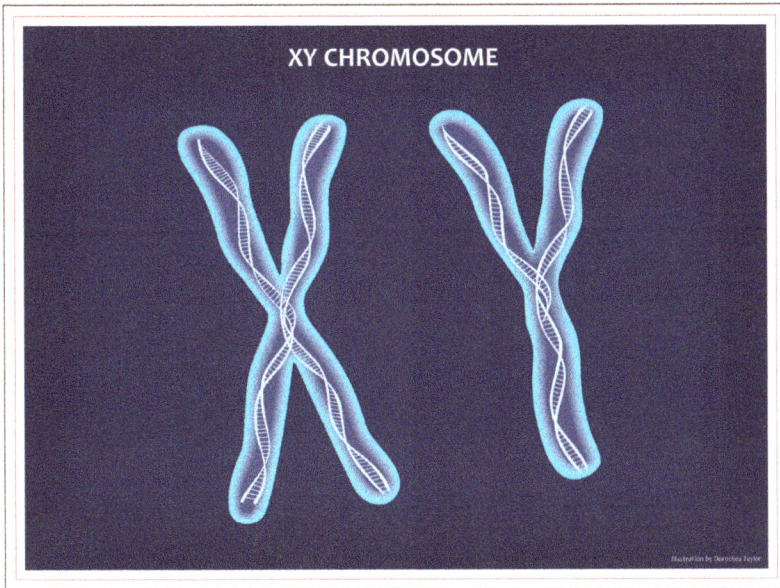

The term chromosome comes from the Greek words for color (chroma) and body (soma). Scientists gave this name to chromosomes because they are cell structures, or bodies, which are strongly stained by some colorful dyes used in research.

What do chromosomes do?

The unique structure of chromosomes keeps DNA tightly wrapped around spool-like proteins, called histones. Without such packaging, DNA molecules would be too long to fit inside cells. For example, if all of the DNA molecules in a single human cell were unwound from their histones and placed end-to-end, they would stretch 6 feet. For an organism to grow and function properly, cells must constantly divide to produce new cells to replace old, worn-out cells.

During cell division, it is essential that DNA remains intact and evenly distributed among cells. Chromosomes are a key part of the process that ensures DNA is accurately copied and distributed in the vast majority of cell divisions. Still, mistakes do occur on rare occasions.

How many chromosomes do humans have?

Humans have 23 pairs of chromosomes, for a total of 46 chromosomes.

In fact, each species of plants and animals has a set number of chromosomes. A fruit fly, for example, has four pairs of chromosomes, while a rice plant has 12 and a dog, 39. Through the process of fertilization, egg and sperm join to make a cell with 46 chromosomes, called a zygote.

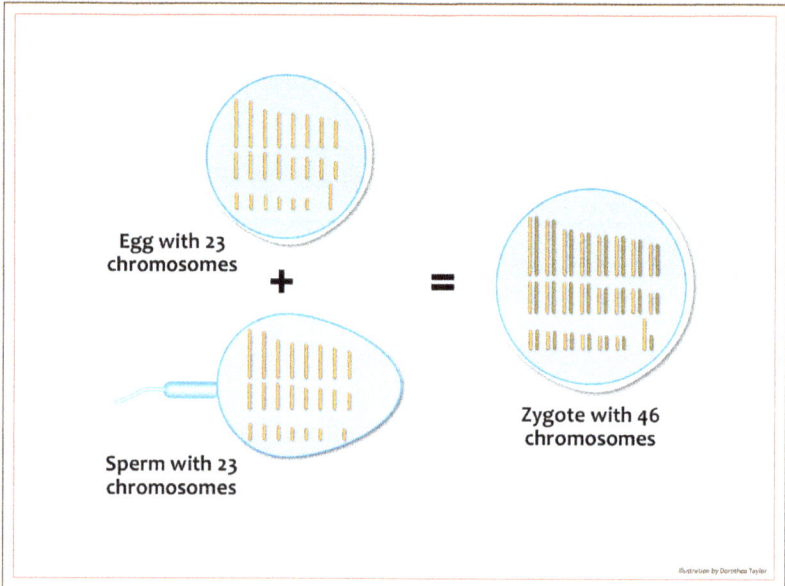

Egg with 23 chromosomes
+
=
Sperm with 23 chromosomes
Zygote with 46 chromosomes

Illustration by Dorothea Taylor

How are chromosomes inherited?

In humans and most other complex organisms, one copy of each chromosome is inherited from the female parent and the other from the male parent. This explains why children inherit some of their traits from their mother and others from their father.

The pattern of inheritance is different for the small circular chromosome found in mitochondria. Only egg cells – and not sperm cells – keep their mitochondria during fertilization. So, mitochondrial DNA is always inherited from the female parent. In humans, a few conditions, including some forms of hearing impairment and diabetes, have been associated with DNA found in the mitochondria.

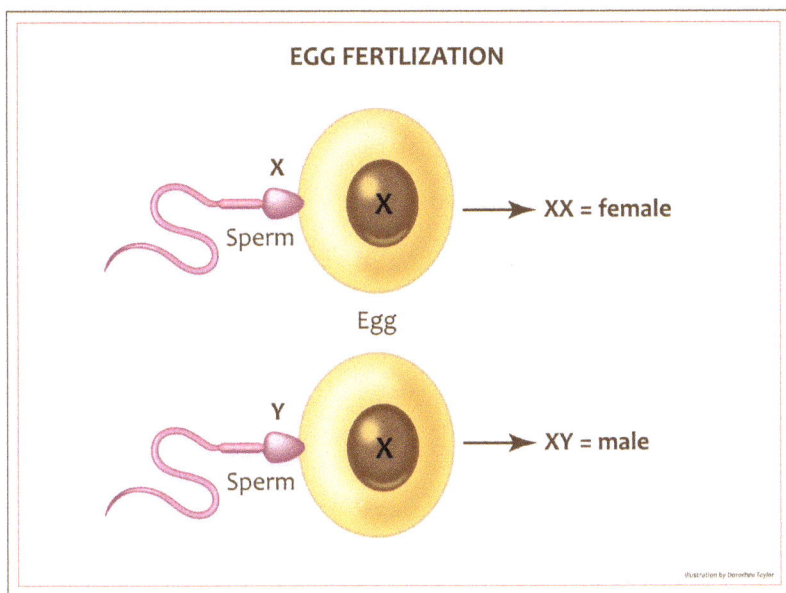

EGG FERTLIZATION

X
Sperm

X

XX = female

Egg

Y
Sperm

X

XY = male

Illustration by Dorothea Taylor

Do males have different chromosomes than females?

Yes, they differ in a pair of chromosomes known as the sex chromosomes. Females have two X chromosomes in their cells, while males have one X and one Y chromosome. Inheriting too many or not enough copies of sex chromosomes can lead to serious problems. For example, females who have extra copies of the X chromosome are usually taller than average and some have mental retardation. Males with more than one X chromosome have Klinefelter syndrome, which is a condition characterized by tall stature and, often, impaired fertility. Another syndrome caused by imbalance in the number of sex chromosomes is Turner syndrome. Women with Turner have one X chromosome only. They are noticeably short, usually do not undergo puberty and some may have kidney or heart problems.

Do all living things have the same types of chromosomes?

Chromosomes vary in number and shape among living things. Most bacteria have one or two circular chromosomes. Humans, along with other animals and plants, have linear chromosomes that are arranged in pairs within the nucleus of the cell. The only human cells that do not contain pairs of chromosomes are reproductive cells, or gametes, which carry just one copy of each chromosome. When two reproductive cells unite, they become a single cell that contains two copies of each chromosome.

This cell then divides, and its successors divide numerous times, eventually producing a mature individual with a full set of paired chromosomes in all its cells. Besides the linear chromosomes found in the nucleus, the cells of humans and other complex organisms carry a much smaller type of chromosome similar to those seen in bacteria. This circular chromosome is found in mitochondria, which are structures located outside the nucleus that serve as the cell's powerhouses.

References:

Alonso, L. & Fuchs, E. (2006) The hair cycle, Journal of Cell Science, issue 119, (pp. 391-393)

Ammann, P., Laib, A., Bonjour, J.-P., Meyer, J. M., Ruegsegger, P. & Rizzoli, R. (2002) Dietary essential aminoacid supplements increase the bone strength by influencing bone mass & bone microarchitecture in an iscaloric low-protein diet, Journal of Bone and Mineral Research, Volume 17, issue 7, (pp. 1264-1272)

Bowtell, .L., Gelly, K., Jackman, M.L., Patel, A., Simeoni, M. & rennie, M.J. (1999) Effect of oral glutamine on whole body carbohydrate storage during recovery from exhaustive exercise, Journal of Applied Physiology, Volume 86, issue 6, (pp. 1770-1777)

DAK-Studie: Immer mehr Senioren mit Mangelernahrung in Klinik, Hamburger Abendblatt (December 2011)

De Angelis, Lissa G. and Siple, Molly (1999). SOS for PMS WHOLE-FOOD SOLUTIONS for PREMENSTRUAL SYNDROME

Dr. Atkin's Vita-Nutrient Solution – Dr. Robert C. Atkins, M.D.

Erdmann, R. & Jones, M., (1987) The Amino Revolution, First Fireside Edition, p2.

Escott-Stump S., eds. Nutrition and diagnosis-Related Care. 6th ed. Philadelphia Pa: Lippincott Williams & Wilkins; 2008.

Evangeliou, A. & Vlassopoulos, D. (2003) Carnitine Metabolism and Deficit – When Supplementation is Necessary?, Current Pharmaceutical Biotechnology, Volume 4, issue 3, (pp. 211-219)

Haneke, E. & Baran, R. (2011) Micronutrients for Hair and Nails, Nutrition for healthy skin, Volume 2, (pp. 149-163)

Hausman, Robert E.; Cooper, Geoffrey M. (2004). The cell: a molecular approach. Washington, D.C: ASM Press. P. 51. ISBN 0-87893-214-3.

Lavie, L., Hafetz, A., Luboshitzky, R. & Lavie, P. (2003) Plasma levels of nitric oxide and L-arginine in sleep apnea patients, Journal of Molecular Neuroscience, Volume 21, issue 1, (pp. 57-63)

Merimee, T.J., Lillicrap, D.A. & Rabinowitz, D. (1965) Effect of arginine on serum-levels of human growth-hormone Lancet, Volume 2, issue 7414, (pp. 668-670)

Michael T. Murray and Joseph E. Pizzorno, authors of "The Encyclopedia of Healing Foods.

Muller, D.M., Seim, H., Kiess, W., Loster, H. & Richter, T. (2002) Effects of Oral l-Carnitine Supplementation on In Vivo Long-Chain Fatty Acid Oxidation in Healthy Adults Metabolism, Volume 51, issue 11, (pp. 1389-1391)

Pookrum, Jewel (1999). Vitamins & Minerals from a to Z

Pookrum, Jewel (2010). STRAIGHT FROM THE HEART A PHYSICIAN'S LOVING MESSAGE OF HEALING & WELLNESS

Power, R.A., Hulver, M. W., Zhang, J. Y., Dubois, J., Marchand, R.M., Ilkayeva, O., Muoio, D.M. & Mynatt, R.L. (2007) Carnitine revisited: potential use as adjunctive treatment Diabetes Diabetologia, Volume 50, issue 4, (pp. 824-832)

Piatti, P.M., Monti, L.D., Valsecchi, G., Magni, F., Setola, E., Marchesi, F., Galli-Kienle, M., Pozza, G. & Alberti, K.G.M.M. (2001) Long-term oral L-arginine administration improves peripheral and hepatic insulin sensitivity in type 2 diabetic patients, Diabetes Care, Volume 24, issue 5, (pp. 875-880)

Prada, P.O., Hirabara, S.M., de Souza, C.T., Schenka, A.A., Zecchin,

H.G., Vassallo, J., Velloso, L.A., Carneiro, E., carvalheira, J.B., Curi, R. & Saad, M.J. (2007) L-glutamine supplementation induces insulin resistance in adipose tissue and improves insulin signaling in liver and muscle with diet-induced obesity, Diabetologia, Volume 50, issue 9, (pp. 149-159)

Prescription for Nutritional Healing – James F. Balch, M.D., and Phyllis A. Balch, C.N.C. –

1990 – Garden City Park, New Jersey: Avery Publishing.

Soeken, K.L., Lee, W.L., Bausell, R.B., Agelli, M. & Berman, B.M. (2002) Safety and efficacy of S-adenosylmethionine (SAMe) for osteoarthritis, Journal of Family Practice, Volume 51, (pp. 425-430)

The Doctor's Vitamin and Mineral Encyclopedia – Simon Saul Hendler, M.D., Ph.D. (New York, New York: Simon and Schuster, 1990).

The Healing Nutrients Within Facts, Finding and New Research on Amino Acids –

- Eric R. Braverman, M.D.
- "The Illustrated Encyclopedia of Healing Remedies"; Norman Shealy 1998
- "Wise Woman Herbal for the Childbearing Year"; Susun Weed; 1986.
- "The Yoga of Herbs"; David Frawley and Vasant Lad; 2001
- 1. http://natural-fertility-info.com/american-ginseng-male-fertility-tonic.html

  2. http://natural-fertility-info.com/tribulus-fertility.html

  3. http://natural-fertility-info.com/maca

  4. http://natural-fertility-info.com/saw-palmetto-fertility.html

  5. Tenny, Deanne. Yohimbe, Woodland Publishing, 1997.

The Latest Advances in Sports Nutrition – Tara Watkins – Vitamin Retailer, November 1995, p. 42-49.

The Latest Advances in Sports Nutrition – Tara Watkins – Vitamin Retailer, November 1995, p. 42-49.

The New York Public Library SCIENCE DESK REFERENCE (1995).

Toda, N., Ayajiki, K. & Okamura, T. (2005) Nitric oxide and penile erectile function, Pharmacol Ther., Volume 106, issue 2, (pp. 233-266)

Trumbo P, Schlicker S, Yates AA, Poos M; Food and Nutrition Board of the Institute of Medicine, The National Academies. Dietary reference intakes for energy, carbohydrate, fiber, fat, fatty acids, cholesterol, protein, and amino acids. J Am Diet Assoc. 2002;102(11):1621-1630.

Watanabe F, Katsura H, Takenaka S, Fujita T, Abe K, Tamura Y, Nakatsuka T, Nakano Y. Pseudo vitamin B(12) is the predominant carbamide of an algal health food, spirulina tablets. J Agric Food Chem. 1999 Nov;47(11):4736-41.

Welbourne, T.C. (1995) Increased plasma bicarbonate and growth hormone after an oral glutamine load, The American Journal of Clinical Nutrition, Volume 61, issue 5, (pp.1058-1061)

Williams, J.Z., Abumrad, N. & Barbul, A. (2002) Effect of a Specialized Amino Acid Mixture on Human Collagen Deposition, Annals of Surgery, Volume 236, issue 3, (pp. 369-375)

Wu, G.A.B., Meininger, C.J., Knabe, D.A., Baze, F.W.A. & Rhoads, J.M. (2000) Arginine nutrition in development, health and disease, Current Opinion in Clinical Nutrition & Metabolic Care, Volume 3, issue 1, (pp. 59-66)

http://www.amymyersmd.com/2016/04/digestive-enzymes/

http://blog.kulikulifoods.com/2015/12/13/case-study-moringa-the-amino-acids-depot/

http://www.babyboomerfitnessusa.com/minerals.html

https://beautyhealthtips.in/minerals-essential-for-your-body-and-mind/

www.caoh.org/vitamins.html

http://doctor.ndtv.com/photodetail/ndtv/page/2/id/7286/stage_ of pregnancy_-_month_by_month.html

http://facts.randomhistory.com/random-facts-about-menstruation.html

https://www.genome.gov/26524120/chromosomes-fact-sheet/

https://www.google.com/search?q=menstrual+cycle+chart&rlz=1C1PRFC_enUS566US567&tbm=isch&tbo=u&source=univ&sa=X&ved=0ahUKEwimtZmhrJvUAhWBKiYKHRa-OC0MQsAQIIw&biw=1366&bih=638#imgrc=XkCf50aEWE_ebM:

https://www.healthaliciousness.com

http://healthyeating.sfgate.com/vitamins-menstrual-cycle-8811.html

www.kirkwood.k12.mo.us/parent_student/KHS/ricejul/.../MenstrualCyclePPT.pdf

http://medical-dictionary.thefreedictionary.com/anus

http://medical-dictionary.thefreedictionary.com/dysbiosis

https://medlineplus.gov/ency/article/002222.htm

www.nlm.nih.gov/midlineplus/druginfo/natural/964.html

http://www.onegreenplanet.org/natural-health/need-protein-amino-acids-found-abundantly-in-plants/

https://www.prebiotin.com/prebiotin-academy/what-are-prebiotics/prebiotics-vs-probiotics/

http://qwcli.org/bio-feedback

http://www.webmd.com/sex-relationships/guide/male-reproductive-system?page=2

http://williams.medicine.wisc.edu/aminoacidcodes.pdf

GLOSSARY

REPRODUCTIVE SYSTEM

"**Abdomen [ab-dōm·ən** *or* **ab·də,mən]** — The abdomen (commonly called the belly) is the body space between the thorax (chest) and pelvis. The diaphragm forms the upper surface of the abdomen. At the level of the pelvic bones, the abdomen ends, and the pelvis begins. The abdomen contains all the digestive organs, including the stomach, small and large intestines, pancreas, liver, and gallbladder. These organs are held together loosely by connecting tissues (mesentery) that allow them to expand and to slide against each other. The abdomen also contains the kidneys and spleen. Many important blood vessels travel through the abdomen, including the aorta, inferior vena cava, and dozens of their smaller branches. In the front, the abdomen is protected by a thin, tough layer of tissue called fascia. In front of the fascia are the abdominal muscles and skin. In the rear of the abdomen are the back muscles.

Abstinence [ab-ste-nens] — Not having any type of intercourse or sex play with a partner. Abstinence is the only birth control method that is 100% effective in preventing pregnancy as well as sexually transmitted diseases. Being abstinent includes the practice of voluntarily refraining from some or all aspects of sexual activity.

Amenorrhea [ā,menə'rēə] – The absence of menstrual periods. Primary amenorrhea is the failure to start having a period by the age of 16.

Amniotic Fluid [am-ne-ot-ik] [floo-id] – The amniotic sac is filled with the amniotic fluid. This sac is your baby's home, gymnasium, and protection from outside knocks, bumps, and other external pressures. The amniotic sac allows the fetus ample room to swim and move around which helps build muscle tone. To keep the baby cozy, the amniotic sac and fluid maintain a slightly higher temperature than the mother's body, usually 99.7 F. At week 10, there is around 30 ml of fluid present. The amniotic fluid will reach its peak around weeks 34-36 at about 1 liter. When your water breaks, it is this sac that ruptures and this fluid that leaves the body. Your baby's life is still being supported by the umbilical cord, and you should be meeting your baby soon!

Anus [ā·nəs] — The anus is the hole in the middle of your buttocks. The lower opening of the digestive tract. It is associated with the anal sphincter and lies in the cleft between the buttocks, through which fecal (poop) matter is extruded.

Birth Control [bûrth] [kon-trol] — Restriction of the number of offspring by means of contraceptive measures, projects, programs, or methods to control reproduction, by either improving or diminishing fertility.

Bladder [bl d r] — A hollow organ in the lower abdomen that stores urine. The kidneys filter waste from the blood and produce urine, which enters the bladder through two tubes, called ureters. Urine leaves the bladder through another tube, the urethra. In women, the urethra is a short tube that opens just in front of the vagina. In men, it is longer, passing through the prostate gland and then the penis. Also known as urinary bladder and vesical.

Bloating [blot] — Is any abnormal general swelling, or increase in diameter of the abdominal area. As a symptom, the patient feels a full and tight abdomen, which may cause abdominal pain, and sometimes accompanied by increased stomach growling or more seriously the total lack of it.

Blood [bluhd] — The "circulating tissue" of the body; the fluid and its suspended formed elements that are circulated through the heart, arteries, capillaries, and veins; blood is the means by which 1) oxygen and nutritive materials are transported to the tissues, and 2) carbon dioxide and various metabolic products are removed for excretion. Blood consists of a pale yellow or gray-yellow fluid, plasma, in which are suspended red blood cells (erythrocytes), white blood cells (leukocytes), and platelets. See also: arterial blood, venous blood.

Body Cavity [bode] [kāv'□-tē] — Any of the spaces in the human body that contain organs.

Breast [brest] — Either of the pair of milk-secreting mammary glands extending from the front of the chest in pubescent and adult human females and some other mammals.

Broad Ligament [brôd] [lig-e-ment] — The broad ligament of the uterus is the wide fold of peritoneum that connects the sides of the uterus to the walls and floor of the pelvis.

Buttocks [but-uk] – In humans, either of the two fleshy protuberances forming the lower and back part of the hips; in animals the rump.

Cervix [sər·viks] — Located between the vagina and uterus, the cervix serves as a passageway for menstrual blood on the way out, and semen on the way in. (During childbirth, the cervix slowly thins and opens, allowing the baby to move from the uterus and into the vaginal canal.) The cervix opens, closes, and changes in texture throughout a woman's menstrual cycle.

Cervical Mucus [sər·və·kəl] [myü·kəs] – A mucus secreted by glands found in and around the cervix, cervical mucus changes in consistency throughout a woman's reproductive cycle. Cervical mucus may also be referred to as cervical fluid. The job of cervical mucus is to either prevent anything from entering the uterus through the cervix (by becoming sticky and thick), or to nourish and help transport sperm through the cervix (by becoming more abundant, stretchy, and closer to the consistency of raw egg white.)

Circumcision [sûr-kəms☐zh`ən] – Is the surgical removal of the foreskin, the tissue covering the head of the penis. It is an ancient practice that has its origin in religious rites. Today, many parents have their sons circumcised for religious or other reasons. Circumcision is usually performed on the first or second day after birth. During a circumcision, the foreskin is freed from the head of the penis (glans), and the excess foreskin is clipped off. If done in the newborn period, the procedure takes about five to 10 minutes. Adult circumcision takes about one hour. The circumcision heals in five to seven days.

Clitoris [klit-er-is, kli-tôr-is] — A small erectile female organ located within the anterior junction of the labia minora that develops from the same embryonic mass of tissue as the penis and is responsive to sexual stimulation.

Conception [kon-sep-shen] – The act of becoming pregnant; fertilization of an ovum by a spermatozoon. The entity formed by the union of the male sperm and female ovum; an embryo or zygote.

Condom [kon-dom] — A flexible sheath, usually made of thin rubber or latex, designed to cover the penis during sexual intercourse for contraceptive purposes or as a means of preventing sexually transmitted diseases. Condoms were originally used as a contraceptive to prevent unwanted pregnancies. A similar device, consisting of a loose-fitting polyurethane sheath closed at one end that is inserted intravaginally before sexual intercourse. Also known as a "rubber."

Connective Tissue Layer [k*uh*-nek-tiv] [tish-oo] [ley-er] – A material made up of fibers forming a framework and support structure for body tissues and organs.

Constipation [kon-ste-pa-shon] — Abnormally delayed or infrequent passage of dry hardened feces.

Contraception [käntrə'sepSHən] — The deliberate use of artificial methods or other techniques to prevent pregnancy as a consequence of sexual intercourse. The major forms of artificial contraception are barrier methods, of which the most common is the condom; the contraceptive pill, which contains synthetic sex hormones that prevent ovulation in the female; intrauterine devices, such as the coil, which prevent the fertilized ovum from implanting in the uterus; and male or female sterilization.

Corpus Luteum [kawr-p*uh*s loo-tee-*uh*m] — A yellow mass of cells that forms from a mature ovarian follicle after ovulation and that secretes progesterone. If fertilization of the egg occurs, the corpus luteum persists for the first few months of pregnancy.

Cowper's Fluid [kou-pers] [floo-id] — Pre-ejaculate (also known as pre-ejaculatory fluid, preseminal fluid, or Cowper's fluid, and colloquially as pre-cum) is the clear, colorless, viscous fluid that emits from the urethra of a man's penis when he is sexually aroused. It is similar in composition to semen, but has some significant chemical differences. The fluid is discharged during arousal, masturbation, foreplay or at an early stage during sex, sometime before the man fully reaches orgasm and semen is ejaculated. It is primarily produced by the bulbourethral glands (Cowper's glands) with the glands of Littre (the mucus-secreting urethral glands) also contributing. Pre-ejaculate contains some chemicals associated with semen.

Cowper's Gland (Bulbourethral Glands) [kou-pers] [¦bəl·bō·yu′rēth·rəl ,gland] — Also called Cowper's glands, these are pea-sized structures located on the sides of the urethra just below the prostate gland. These glands produce a clear, slippery fluid that empties directly into the urethra. This fluid serves to lubricate the urethra and to neutralize any acidity that may be present due to residual drops of urine in the urethra.

Craving [kra-ving] — An intense, urgent, or abnormal desire or longing.

Diarrhea [di-e-re—e] — Abnormally frequent intestinal evacuations with more or less fluid stools (poop, feces). Diarrhea occurs because more fluid passes through the large intestine (colon) than that organ can absorb.

Dysmenorrhea [dismenə'rēə] — Painful menstruation, typically involving abdominal cramps.

Ectopic Pregnancy [ec-to-pe-c] [preg-nen-se] — An ectopic pregnancy (EP) is a condition in which a fertilized egg settles and grows in any location other than the inner lining of the uterus. The vast majority of ectopic pregnancies are so-called tubal pregnancies and occur in the Fallopian tube (98%); however, they can occur in other locations, such as the ovary, cervix, and abdominal cavity. An ectopic pregnancy occurs in about one in 50 pregnancies. A molar differs from an ectopic in that it is usually a mass of tissue derived from an egg with incomplete genetic information that grows in the uterus in a grape-like mass that can cause symptoms to those of pregnancy.

Eggs [eg] — Every woman is born with eggs which, when fertilized, develop into a baby. At birth, women have about 1 million of these eggs stored in their ovaries. By the time you start menstruating, you have about 400 000 eggs available for fertilization. Over time, the number of eggs that you have in your ovaries will decline, and you may not release an egg every month. Eventually, as you enter menopause, your body will only have a few hundred eggs left and you will probably not ovulate again due to a change in your hormone levels.

Ejaculation [i,jak·yə-lā·shən] — Is the ejection of semen (usually carrying sperm) from the male reproductive tract, and is usually accompanied by orgasm. It is usually the final stage and natural objective of male sexual stimulation, and an essential component of natural conception.

Embryo [em-bre-o] – An organism in the initial stages of development within the womb.

Endocrine System [en-do-krin, -kren, -krin] [sis-tem] — It influences almost every cell, organ, and function of our bodies. The endocrine system is instrumental in regulating mood, growth and development, tissue function, metabolism, and sexual function and reproductive processes. The foundations of the endocrine system are the hormones and glands.

Endometriosis [endō,mētrē'ōsis] — a condition resulting from the appearance of endometrial tissue outside the uterus and causing pelvic pain. Endometrium Uterine Lining [en-do-me-tre-om] [yoo-ter-in [lahyning] – The mucous membrane that lines the uterus; thickens under hormonal control and if pregnancy does not occur, is sheds in menstruation, if pregnancy does occur sheds with the placenta in at parturition.

Epididymis [ep·ə-did·ə·məs] — The epididymis is a long, coiled tube that rests on the backside of each testicle. It transports and stores sperm cells that are produced in the testes. It also is the job of the epididymis to bring the sperm to maturity, since the sperm that emerge from the testes are immature and incapable of fertilization. During sexual arousal, contractions force the sperm into the vas deferens.

Epithelium [ep-*uh*-thee-lee-*uh*m] – Tissue that covers a surface, or lines a cavity or the like, and that, in addition, performs any of various secretory, transporting, or regulatory functions.

Estrogen [estrəjən] — A female steroid hormone that is produced by the ovaries and, in lesser amounts, by the adrenal cortex, placenta, and male testes. Estrogen helps control and guide sexual development, including the physical changes associated with puberty. It also influences the course of ovulation in the monthly menstrual cycle, lactation after pregnancy, aspects of mood, and the aging process. Production of estrogen changes naturally over the female lifespan, reaching adult levels with the onset of puberty (menarche) and decreasing in middle age until the onset of menopause. Estrogen deficiency can lead to lack of menstruation (amenorrhea), persistent difficulties associated with menopause (such as mood swings and vaginal dryness), and osteoporosis in older age. In cases of estrogen deficiency, natural and synthetic estrogen preparations may be prescribed. Estrogen is also a component of many oral contraceptives. An overabundance of estrogen in men causes development of female secondary sexual characteristics (feminization), such as enlargement of breast tissue.

External Orifice Os [ik-stur-nl] [awr-*uh*-fis] or (Ostium) [os-tee*uh*m] – The vaginal opening of the uterus.

Fallopian Tube [fəl-lō·pē·ən tŭb] — One of the two Fallopian tubes that transport the egg from the ovary to the uterus (the womb). These tubes bear the name of Gabriele Falloppio (also spelled Falloppia), a 16th-century (c. 1523-62) Italian physician and surgeon who was expert in anatomy, physiology, and pharmacology.

Female Reproductive System [fee-meyl] [ree-pr*uh*-duhk-tiv] [sist*uh*m] — Is designed to conduct several functions. It produces the female egg cells necessary for reproduction, called the ova or oocytes. The system is designed to transport the ova to the site of fertilization. Conception, the fertilization of an egg by a sperm, normally occurs in the fallopian tubes. The next step for the fertilized egg is to implant into the walls of the uterus, beginning the initial stages of pregnancy. If fertilization and/or implantation does not take place, the system is designed to menstruate (the monthly shedding of the uterine lining). In addition, the female reproductive system produces female sex hormones that maintain the reproductive cycle.

Fertile [fûr-tl] — Capable of reproducing.

Fertilized [fûr-tl-iz] — The union of male and female gametes to form a zygote.

Fetus [fe-tus] — An unborn offspring, from the embryo stage (the end of the eighth week after conception, when the major structures have formed) until birth.

Follicle Fluid [fol-i-k*uh*l] [floo-id] — A follicle is a fluid-filled sac that contains an immature egg, or oocyte.

Follicle Stimulating Hormone [¦fäl·ə·kəl ¦stim·yə,lād·iŋ hȯr,mōn] — A gonadotropic hormone of the anterior pituitary gland that stimulates the growth of follicles in the ovary and induces the formation of sperm in the testis.

Follicle Stimulating Hormone Releasing Factor (FSH-RF) [fol-ik*uh*l] [stim-y*uh*-leyt-ng] [hawr-mohn] [ree-lees-ng] [fak-ter] — A hormone from the hypothalamus that stimulates the synthesis and release of FSH and luteinizing hormone from the anterior pituitary.

Foreskin (Prepuce) [fôr-skin, fer-] ['prep·əs] — The fold of skin, which covers the head (the glans) of the penis. Also called the prepuce.

Fundus [fuhn-d*uh*s] — The upper rounded extremity of the uterus above the openings of the fallopian tubes.

Gametes ['gæmiːt gə'miːt] — Gametes are reproductive cells that unite during sexual reproduction to form a new cell called a zygote. In humans, male gametes are sperm and female gametes are ova (eggs). Sperm are motile and have a long, tail-like projection called a flagellum. Ova, however, are non-motile and large in comparison to the male gamete. Gametes are produced by a type of cell division called meiosis. They are haploid, meaning that they contain only one set of chromosomes. When the haploid male and female gametes unite in a process called fertilization, they form what is called a zygote. The zygote is diploid and contains two sets of chromosomes.

Glans [glanz] — Small rounded body or gland-like mass, such as the head of the penis (glans penis) or clitoris.

Genitalia [jen-i-tale-e, -tal-ye] — The sexual organs of reproduction, especially the external organs. Such as the testicles and penis of a male; and the labia, clitoris and vagina of a female.

Gestation [je'stāSHən] — The process of carrying or being carried in the womb between conception and birth.

Gonadotropin-Releasing Hormone Family [go-nad-o-tro-pin-riles-ing] [hor-mōn] — Are a family of peptides that play a pivotal role in reproduction. The main function of GnRH is to act on the pituitary to stimulate the synthesis and secretion of luteinizing and follicle-stimulating hormones, but GnRH also acts on the brain, retina, sympathetic nervous system, gonads, and placenta in certain species. There seems to be at least three forms GnRH. The second form is expressed in midbrain and seems to be widespread. The third form has been found so far only in fish. GnRH s a C-terminal amidated decapeptide processed from a larger precursor protein. Four of the ten residues are perfectly conserved in all species where GnRH has been sequenced.

Hormones [hôr-mon] — As the body's chemical messengers, **hormones** transfer information and instructions from one set of cells to another. Many different hormones move through the bloodstream, but each type of hormone is designed to affect only certain cells.

Human Chorionic Gonadotropin (hCG) [hyoo-mun] [kôr-e-on, kor-][go-na-do-tropin, -trop-in] — hCG is a hormone produced during pregnancy.

Hypothalamus [hi-po-thal-e-mus] — A region of the brain, between the thalamus and the midbrain, that functions as the main control center for the autonomic nervous system by regulating sleep cycles, body temperature, appetite, etc. And function as an endocrine gland by producing hormones, including the releasing factors that control the hormonal secretions of the pituitary gland.

Infertile [-In-fûr-tl] — Absent or diminished fertility. The persistent inability to conceive a child.

Internal Orifice [in-tur-nl] [awr-*uh*-fis, orInternal (Ostium) [os-tee*uh*m] — The internal opening of the cervical canal.

Labia Majora [labe-e] [me-jôr-e, -jor-e] — The two outer rounded folds of adipose tissue that lie on either side of the vaginal opening and that form the external lateral boundaries of the vulva.

Labia Minora [la-be-e] [me-nôr-e, -nor-e] — The inner folds of skin of the external female genitalia.

Labioscrotal [la-bis-cro-tal] — Relating to or being a swelling or ridge on each side of the embryonic rudiment of the penis or clitoris, which develops into one of the scrotal sacs in the male and one of the labia majora in the female.

Luteinizing Hormone (LH) [lüd-ē-ə,nīz-iŋ hôr,mōn] — LH is a hormone secreted by the pituitary gland. It, along with FSH, helps a woman's egg mature and develop. There is a surge of LH right before ovulation that triggers the egg's release from the ovary, and this surge is what at-home ovulation predictor kits look for. In men, LH engages in the production of testosterone, which in turn affects sperm cell growth and development.

Luteinizing Hormone Releasing Factor (LH-RF) ['lüd-ē-ə,nīz-iŋ 'hôr,mōn] — Produced by the anterior lobe of the pituitary gland that stimulates ovulation and the development of the corpus luteum in the female and the production of testosterone by the interstitial cells of the testis in the male.

Male Reproductive System [meyl] [ree-pr*uh*-duhk-tiv] [sis-t*uh*m] — The entire male reproductive system is dependent on hormones, which are chemicals that regulate the activity of many diverse types of cells or organs. The primary hormones involved in the male reproductive system are follicle-stimulating hormone, luteinizing hormone, and testosterone. Most of the male reproductive system is located outside of the body. These external structures include the penis, scrotum, and testicles.

Follicle-stimulating hormone is necessary for sperm production (spermatogenesis), and luteinizing hormone stimulates the production of testosterone, which is also needed to make sperm. Testosterone is responsible for the development of male characteristics, including muscle mass and strength, fat distribution, bone mass, facial hair growth, voice change, and sex drive.

Menarche [men͵ärkē] – The time in a girl's life when menstruation first begins. During the menarche period, menstruation may be irregular and unpredictable. Also known as female puberty.

Menorrhagia [menə'rāj(ē)ə] – Abnormally heavy bleeding at menstruation.

Menstruation (Menses) [men-stroo-a-shen] [men-sez] – Menstruation is the vaginal bleeding that occurs in adolescent girls and women as a result of hormonal changes. It normally happens in a predictable pattern, once a month. Menstruation is part of the menstrual cycle, which helps a woman's body prepare for the possibility of pregnancy each month. The parts of the body involved in the menstrual cycle include the uterus and cervix, the ovaries, fallopian tubes, the brain and pituitary gland, and the vagina. Certain body chemicals known as hormones rise and fall during the month, causing the menstrual cycle to occur.

Menstrual Cramps [men-stroo-el] [kramp] – Menstrual pain, or menstrual cramps, are caused by the contraction of the uterus. Low abdominal pain that may range from a colicky feeling to a constant dull ache. For these girls, the pain brings aches in the lower back, the abdomen, the pelvic area, and sometimes even in the upper thighs. Fortunately, most menstrual discomfort is normal, but there are times when the pain can be associated with disease or other gynecological problems. The pain may radiate to the lower back and legs. Menstrual cramps are often associated with the beginning of menses, reaching a peak in 24 hours, and subsiding after 2 days.

Menstrual Cycle [men-stroo-el] [si-kel] – The word menstruation (say men-strew-ay-shun) comes from a Latin word 'mens,' which means month. The monthly cycle of changes in the ovaries and the lining of the uterus (endometrium), starting with the preparation of an egg for fertilization. When the follicle of the prepared egg in the ovary breaks, it is released for fertilization and ovulation occurs. Unless pregnancy occurs, the cycle ends with the shedding of part of the endometrium, which is menstruation.

Although it is actually the end of the physical cycle, the first day of menstrual bleeding is designated as "day 1" of the menstrual cycle in medical parlance.

Mitochondria [mite-kon-dre-a] — Mitochondria are self-replicating organelles that play a significant role in generating energy for the cell. They are therefore, called powerhouse of the cell.

Newborn [noo-bawrn] — An infant (from the Latin word *infans*, meaning "unable to speak" or "speechless") is the very young offspring of a human or other mammal. When applied to humans, the term is usually considered synonymous with baby, but the latter is commonly applied to the young of any animal. When a human child learns to walk, the term *toddler* may be used instead.

Oligomenorrhea [ol-i-gō-men-ō-rē-ă] — In frequent or exceptionally light menstruation. With oligomenorrhea, menstrual periods occur at intervals of greater than 35 days, with only four to nine periods in a year.

Orgasm [ȯr,gaz·əm] — An orgasm is the intense feeling of physical pleasure that human beings experience at the climax of sexual stimulation. It is the climax of sexual excitement, experienced as an intensely pleasurable sensation caused by a series of strong involuntary contractions of the muscles of the genital organs. Both men and women can have an orgasm: men need to orgasm to deposit sperm near the cervix; but women do not necessarily need an orgasm to get pregnant.

Ovary [ōv·ə·rē] — One of two female reproductive organs. In women, ovaries are almond-sized organs located in the pelvis, within a fibrous band next to the uterus. Their purpose is to produce and release eggs for fertilization. Ovaries produce sex hormones such as estrogen, progesterone and, in lesser amounts, testosterone. During menopause, the ovaries become less and less active, although they continue to produce some hormones well beyond the end of menses.

Oviduct [oh-vi-duhkt] (Fallopian Tubes) — Transport the egg from an ovary to the uterus (womb).

Ovulation [,äv·yə-lā-shən] — Ovulation refers to that time when your ovary releases an egg for fertilization. It happens once a month and is a distinct stage of your menstrual cycle. Usually, one egg is released from your ovary about two weeks before you expect your period. For most women with a 28-

day cycle, ovulation occurs on or around the 14th day. Some women have shorter or longer cycles, ranging anywhere from 21 to 35 days. Ovulation usually occurs sooner if you have a short cycle and later if you have a long cycle. Ovulation is regulated by special hormones that are released by various parts of your body. Your brain contains hormones that stimulate the growth and development of your eggs. Your ovaries contain female sex hormones like estrogen and progesterone, which help to release eggs during ovulation. It is the interplay between these hormones that triggers ovulation and menstruation. The ovulation cycle is dependent upon signals sent by your body. These signals are sent in the form of changing hormone levels; as your hormone levels increase and decrease, your body responds by triggering separate phases of your menstrual cycle. Ovulation is dependent on signals sent from three main parts of your body:

- the hypothalamus (found in the brain)
- the pituitary gland (found at the base of the brain, near the spine)
- the ovaries (located on either side of your uterus)

Penis [pe-nis] — This is the male organ used in sexual intercourse. Male sex organ, which also provides the channel for urine to leave the body. It has three parts: the root, which attaches to the wall of the abdomen; the body, or shaft; and the glans, which is the cone-shaped part at the end of the penis. The glans, also called the head of the penis, is covered with a loose layer of skin called foreskin. This skin is sometimes removed in a procedure called circumcision. The opening of the urethra, the tube that transports semen and urine, is at the tip of the penis. The penis also contains a number of sensitive nerve endings. The body of the penis is cylindrical in shape and consists of three circular shaped chambers. These chambers are made up of special, sponge-like tissue. This tissue contains thousands of large spaces that fill with blood when the man is sexually aroused. As the penis fills with blood, it becomes rigid and erect, which allows for penetration during sexual intercourse. The skin of the penis is loose and elastic to accommodate changes in penis size during an erection.

Parturition [pärCHoŏˈriSHən] — The action of giving birth to young; childbirth.

Pelvic Cavity [pel·vik ¦kav·əd·ē] — The pelvic cavity is a body cavity that is bounded by the bones of the. Its oblique roof is the pelvic inlet (the superior opening of the pelvis). Its lower boundary is the pelvic floor. The pelvic cavity primarily contains reproductive organs, the urinary bladder, the pelvic colon, and the rectum.

Pelvis [pel·vəs] — Structure shaped like a funnel in the outlet of the kidney into which urine is discharged before passing into the ureter.

Phallus [fal·əs] — The penis, the clitoris, or the sexually undifferentiated embryonic organ out of which either of these develops.

Phytoestrogen [fītō'estrəjən] — An estrogen occurring naturally in legumes, considered beneficial in some diets.

Pituitary Gland [pi-too-i-ter-e, -tyoo-] [gland] — A small oval endocrine gland attached to the base of the vertebrate brain and consisting of an anterior and a posterior lobe, the secretions of which control the other endocrine glands and influence growth, metabolism, and maturation.

Placenta [ple-sen-te] — The placenta has been described as a pancake-shaped organ that attaches to the inside of the uterus and is connected to the fetus by the umbilical cord. The placenta produces pregnancy-related hormones, including chorionic gonadotropin (hCG), estrogen, and progesterone. The placenta is responsible for working as a trading post between the mother's and the baby's blood supply. Small blood vessels carrying the fetal blood run through the placenta, which is full of maternal blood. Nutrients and oxygen from the mother's blood are transferred to the fetal blood, while waste products are transferred from the fetal blood to the maternal blood, without the two blood supplies mixing.

Pregnancy [preg·nən·sē] — Process of human gestation that takes place in the female's body as a fetus develops, from fertilization to birth (*see* parturition). It begins when a viable sperm from the male and egg from the ovary merge in the fallopian tube (*see* fertilized). The fertilized egg (zygote) grows by cell division as it moves toward the uterus, where it implants in the lining and grows into an embryo and then a fetus. A placenta and umbilical cord develop for nutrient and waste exchange between the circulations of mother and fetus. A protective fluid-filled amniotic sac encloses and cushions the fetus.

Premenstrual Syndrome (PMS) [pre-men-stroo-el] [sin-drom] — Has a wide variety of symptoms, including mood swings, tender breasts, food cravings, fatigue, irritability, and depression. An estimated 3 of every 4 menstruating women experience some form of premenstrual syndrome.

These problems tend to peak during your late 20s and early 30s. Symptoms tend to recur in a predictable pattern. Yet the physical and emotional changes you experience with premenstrual syndrome may be particularly intense in some months and only slightly noticeable in others.

Progesterone [pro-jes-te-ron] – A female hormone, the principal hormone that prepares the uterus to receive and sustain fertilized eggs. A steroid hormone, $C21H30O2$, secreted by the corpus luteum of the ovary and by the placenta, which acts to prepare the uterus for implantation of the fertilized ovum, to maintain pregnancy, and to promote development of the mammary glands. Progesterone levels increase in the second half of the menstrual cycle, after ovulation, and usually remain high if the woman gets pregnant. Progesterone helps to maintain the lining of the uterus in order to support a pregnancy.

Prostate Gland [pros-tat] [gland] – The prostate gland is a walnut-sized structure that is located below the urinary bladder in front of the rectum. The prostate gland contributes additional fluid to the ejaculate. Prostate fluids also help to nourish the sperm. The urethra, which carries the ejaculate to be expelled during orgasm, runs through the center of the prostate gland.

Puberty ['pju:bəti] – Puberty is a normal phase of development that occurs when a child's body transitions into an adult body and readies for the possibility of reproduction. The period or age at which a person is first capable of sexual reproduction of offspring. Physical signs that a girl is entering puberty include growth spurts, breast development, underarm and pubic hair growth, facial acne, body odor, and menstruation. Physical signs that a boy is entering puberty include a deepening of the voice, muscle growth, pubic hair growth, acne, underarm growth, growth spurts, adult body odor, growth of testicles and penis, wet dreams, or the ability to ejaculate. It may take 2 to 4 years before your tween's body fully transitions through puberty. Girls traditionally enter puberty earlier than boys, and it is common for girls to begin showing signs as early as age 9. For most girls, menstruation may begin around the ages of 11 or 12. Girls who show signs of puberty before the age of eight are known to have precocious puberty, which is a treatable condition that should be evaluated by her health care provider. For boys, the first signs of puberty are likely to occur around the ages of 11 or 12.

Pubic Bone [py·u·bik] [bon] — One of the three sections of the hipbone; together these two bones form the front of the pelvis.

Rectum [rek·təm] — The rectum is about eight inches long and serves as a warehouse for poop (feces). It hooks up with the sigmoid colon to the north and with the anal canal to the south. The rectum has little shelves in it called transverse folds. These folds help keep stool in place until you are ready to go to the bathroom. When you are ready, stool enters the lower rectum, moves into the anal canal, and then passes through the anus on its way out.

Reproductive System [¦rē·prə-dək·tiv ,sis·təm] — The system of organs and parts which function in reproduction consisting in the male especially of the testes, penis, seminal vesicles, prostate, and urethra and in the female especially of the ovaries, fallopian tubes, uterus, vagina, and vulva.

Sanitary Pads [san-i-ter-e] [pad] — A disposable pad of absorbent material worn to absorb menstrual flow.

Scrotum [skrōd·əm] — This is the loose pouch-like sac of skin that hangs behind and below the penis. It contains the testicles (also called testes), as well as many nerves and blood vessels. The scrotum acts as a "climate control system" for the testes. For normal sperm development, the testes must be at a temperature slightly cooler than body temperature. Special muscles in the wall of the scrotum allow it to contract and relax, moving the testicles closer to the body for warmth or farther away from the body to cool the temperature.

Secrete [si-kret] — To generate and separate (a substance) from cells or bodily fluids.

Semen [sē·mən] — Which contains sperm (reproductive cells), is expelled (ejaculated) through the end of the penis when the man reaches sexual climax (orgasm). When the penis is erect, the flow of urine is blocked from the urethra, allowing only semen to be ejaculated at orgasm.

Seminal Vesicle [sem·ən·əl ves·i·kəl] — The seminal vesicles are sac-like pouches that attach to the vas deferens near the base of the bladder. The seminal vesicles produce a sugar-rich fluid (fructose) that provides sperm with a source of energy to help them move. The fluid of the seminal vesicles makes up most of the volume of a man's ejaculatory fluid, or ejaculate.

Sperm [spərm] — The term sperm is derived from the Greek word (σπέρμα) *sperma* (meaning "seed") and refers to the male reproductive cells.

Spermatogenesis [spər,mad·ə'jen·ə·səs] — The process of male gamete formation including formation of a spermatocyte from a spermatogonium, meiotic division of the spermatocyte, and transformation of the four resulting spermatids into spermatozoa.

Sexual Intercourse (Copulation [kăp·yə'lā·shən] or Coitus [kō·əd·əs]) — The act conducted for procreation or for pleasure in which, typically, the insertion of the male's erect penis into the female's vagina is followed by rhythmic thrusting usually culminating in orgasm.

Tampons [tam-pon] — A plug of absorbent material inserted into a body cavity or wound to check a flow of blood or to absorb secretions, especially one designed for insertion into the vagina during menstruation.

Testicles (Testes) [tes-ti-kel] [tes-tez] — These are oval organs about the size of large olives that lie in the scrotum, secured at either end by a structure called the spermatic cord. Most men have two testes. The testes are responsible for making testosterone, the primary male sex hormone, and for generating sperm. Within the testes are coiled masses of tubes called seminiferous tubules. These tubes are responsible for producing sperm cells.

Testosterone [tes-tăs·tə,rōn] — A "male hormone" — a sex hormone produced by the testes that encourages the development of male sexual characteristics, stimulates the activity of the male secondary sex characteristics, and prevents changes in them following castration. Chemically, testosterone is 17-beta-hydroxy-4-androstene-3-one. Testosterone is the most potent of the naturally occurring androgens. The androgens cause the development of male sex characteristics, such as a deep voice and a beard; they also strengthen muscle tone and bone mass. High levels of testosterone appear to promote good health in men, for example, lowering the risks of high blood pressure and heart attack.

Toxic Shock Syndrome [tok-sik] [shok] [sin-drohm] — Toxic shock syndrome is a severe disease that involves fever, shock, and problems with the function of several body organs. Toxic shock syndrome is caused by a toxin produced by certain types of *Staphylococcus* bacteria. A similar syndrome, called toxic shock-like syndrome (TSLS), can be caused by Streptococcal bacteria. Not all staph or strep infections cause toxic shock syndrome. Although the earliest cases of toxic shock syndrome involved women who were using tampons during their periods (menstruation), today less than half of current cases are associated with such events.

Umbilical Cord [um-bil-i-kel] [kôrd] — Is the lifeline that attaches the placenta to the fetus. The umbilical cord is made up of three blood vessels: two smaller arteries, which carry blood to the placenta and a larger vein, which returns blood to the fetus. It can grow to be 60 cm long, allowing the baby enough cord to safely move around without causing damage to the cord or the placenta. After the baby is born, the cord is cut (something the baby's father may wish to do); the remaining section will heal and form the baby's belly button. During pregnancy, you may find out that the umbilical cord is in a knot or is wrapped around a part of your baby's body. This is common and cannot be prevented, and it usually does not pose any threats to the baby.

Urethra [yə-rē·thrə] — The tube or duct that carries urine from the bladder and out through the penis. Not to be confused with the ureter that carries urine from each kidney to the bladder. In males, it has the additional function of ejaculating semen when the man reaches orgasm. When the penis is erect during sex, the flow of urine is blocked from the urethra, allowing only semen to be ejaculated at orgasm.

Urinary Bladder [yu̇r·ə,ner·ē blad·ər] — The organ that stores urine, which is collected by the kidneys and transferred to the bladder by the ureters. The bladder empties through the urethra, which passes through the prostate gland and then the penis.

Urine [yu̇r·ən] — The liquid-to-semisolid waste matter excreted by the kidneys, in humans being a yellowish, slightly acid, watery fluid.

Ureter [yoo-re-ter, yoor-i-ter] — The tube or duct that carries urine from each kidney to the bladder.

Urogenital [yoor-o-jen-i-tl] — Of, relating to, or involving both the urinary and genital structures and functions.

Uterine Lining yoo-ter-in, -tuh-rahyn] [lahy-ning] – The inner layer of the uterus (womb); the cells that line the womb; endometrium.

Uterus [yoo-ter-uhs] – A hollow, pear-shaped organ that is located in a woman's lower abdomen, between the bladder and the rectum. The narrow lower portion of the uterus is the cervix (the neck of the uterus). The broader upper part is the corpus, which is made up of three layers of tissue. In women of childbearing age, the inner layer (endometrium) of the uterus goes through a series of monthly changes known as the menstrual cycle. Each month, endometrial tissue grows and thickens in preparation to receive a fertilized egg. Menstruation occurs when this tissue is not used, disintegrates, and passes out through the vagina. The middle layer (myometrium) of the uterus is muscular tissue that expands during pregnancy to hold the growing fetus and contracts during labor to deliver the child. The outer layer (parametrium) also expands during pregnancy and contracts thereafter.

Vagina [və-jī·nə] — The vagina is a muscular canal extending from the cervix to the outside of the body. The muscular canal that extends from the cervix to the outside of the body. It is usually 6 to 7 inches in length, and its walls are lined with mucous membrane. It includes two vault like structures: the anterior (front) vaginal fornix and the posterior (rear) vaginal fornix. The cervix protrudes slightly into the vagina, and through a tiny hole in the cervix (the os), sperm make their way toward the internal reproductive organs. The vagina also includes numerous tiny glands that make vaginal secretions. The word "vagina" is a Latin word meaning "a sheath or scabbard," a scabbard into which one might slide and sheath a sword. The "sword" in the case of the anatomic vagina was the penis. Love and war, it would seem, have been connected in the minds of people for millennia.

Vaginal Fornix [vaj-uh-nl] [fawr-niks] – A recess in the upper part of the vagina caused by the protusion of the uterine cervix into the vagina.

Vas Deferens [vas def·ə·rənz] — The vas deferens is a long, muscular tube that travels from the epididymis into the pelvic cavity, to just behind the bladder. The vas deferens transports mature sperm to the urethra, the tube that carries urine or sperm to outside of the body, in preparation for ejaculation.

Vulva [vŭl′və] — The external genital organs of the female, including the labia majora, labia minora, clitoris, and vestibule of the vagina.

Womb [woom] – A hollow muscular organ in the pelvic cavity of females; contains the developing fetus.

X Chromosome [kro-me-som] – A sex chromosome of humans and most mammals that determines femaleness when paired with another X chromosome and that occurs singly in males.

Y Chromosome [kro-me-som] — A Y-chromosome is the sex chromosome found only in males. The two types of sex chromosomes, X and Y, determine the sex of an embryo. Women have two X chromosomes and men have an X and a Y chromosome. Because of this, the sex of the child is determined by which chromosome the male passes down.

Yolk Sac [yok] [sak, sôk] – A structure that develops in the inner cell mass of the embryo and expands into a vesicle with a thick part that becomes the primitive gut and a thin part that grows into the cavity of the chorion. The cells of the extra embryonic mesoderm differentiate to develop endothelium, primitive blood plasma, and hemoglobin. The yolk sac usually disappears during the seventh week of pregnancy.

Yoni [yo-ne] – A term borrowed from India's ancient language, Sanskrit or Devanagari (Skt., divine language). It can be translated by several English concepts (origin, source, womb, female genitals) and is, considered by many, the most respectful word available for naming what in correct language we call vulva (Lat., female genitals, womb) yet which is often (wrongfully) called vagina (Lat., sheath); unless slang is used.

The term yoni heralds from a culture and religion in which women have long been regarded and honored as the embodiment of divine female energy - the goddess known as *Shakti* - and where the female genitals were/are seen as a sacred symbol of the Great Goddess. Because Tantric, and others worship the Divine in the form of a Goddess, the term Yoni has also acquired other, more cosmic meanings, becoming a symbol of the *Universal Womb*, the *Matrix of Generation* and *Source of All*. In short, the universe really is a yoniverse.

Zygote[zi-got] – Is a fertilized egg cell that results from the union of a female gamete (egg, or ovum) with a male gamete (sperm). In the embryonic development of humans and other animals, the zygote stage is brief and is followed by cleavage, when the single cell becomes subdivided into smaller cells. The zygote represents the first stage in the development of a genetically unique organism. The zygote is endowed with genes from two parents, and thus it is diploid (carrying two sets of chromosomes)."

VITAMINS

Vitamin A (Retinol)

Vitamin A can help support a woman's fertility in many ways, most noticeably is that it promotes better cervical fluid. Not only can it help your body to produce more fluid, but the fluid also itself is more nourishing for the sperm and helps them to live longer, allowing for more time to meet the egg. Vitamin A also assists the follicles in maturing properly. Both in the maturation of an egg and then in assisting the follicle in producing the hormones needed to aid the fertilized egg into the uterus. Vitamin A is used for heavy menstrual periods, premenstrual syndrome (PMS), vaginal infections, yeast infections, "lumpy breasts" (fibrocystic breast disease), and to prevent breast cancer.

Vitamin A Food Source: Butternut squash, kale, turnip greens, spinach, green, swiss chard, romaine lettuce, dandelion greens, beet greens, pak choi, pumpkin, cantaloupe, papaya, mango, passionfruit, watermelon, guava, tomatoes, grapefruit, leeks, brussel sprouts, Chinese broccoli, pumpkin, dried apricot, sweet red, yellow, and green peppers, sweet potatoes, Chinese cabbage, bok choy, pecans, chestnuts, and pistachios.

Vitamin B1 (Thiamin)

Vitamin B1 helps convert carbohydrates (Carbohydrates are found in almost all living things and play a critical role in the proper functioning of the immune system, fertilization, pathogenesis, blood clotting, and human development.) into energy and is essential for the functioning of the heart, muscles, and nervous system.

Vitamin B1 Food Source: Fortified breads, pasta, wheat germ, macadamia nuts, sunflower seeds, pumpkin seeds, acorn squash, boysenberries, dates, grapes, grapefruit, guava, mango, orange pineapple, pomegranate, watermelon, loganberries, avocado, green peas, asparagus, navy beans, black beans, soy beans (edamame), brazil nuts, black beans, black-eyed peas, white beans, buckwheat, cashews, chestnuts, flax seed, hazelnuts, peanuts, pecans, quinoa, brown rice, pistachios, rye, spelt, lima beans, okra, French beans, potatoes, and spirulina.

Vitamin B2 (Riboflavin)

Vitamin B2 is needed for normal cell function, growth, and energy production.

Vitamin B2 Food Source: Almonds, avocado, banana, grapes, lychee, mango, mulberries, passion fruit, pomegranate, prickly pear, artichoke, asparagus, bok choy, brussel sprouts, lima beans, mushrooms, pumpkin, spirulina, sweet potato, winter squash, quinoa, rye, buckwheat, oats sesame seeds, beet greens, swiss chard, chestnuts, wheat (durum, hard red, hard white), pinto beans, navy beans, garbanzo beans, fava beans, asparagus, brown mushrooms (crimini), spinach, and soy beans (edamame).

Vitamin B3 (Niacin/Nicotinic Acid)

Vitamin B3 is essential for converting food to energy, assists in the functioning of the digestive system, skin, and nerves.

Vitamin B3 Food Source: Spirulina, seaweed, chia seeds, peanut butter, paprika, green peas, sunflower seeds, avocado, broccoli, asparagus, kidney beans, bell peppers, tahini, fortified cereal, shitake and portabella mushrooms, boysenberries, loganberries, lychee, mango, peach, passion fruit, artichoke, dates, guava, butternut squash, mushrooms, okra, parsnip, peas, potatoes, spaghetti squash, pumpkin, spirulina, barley, buckwheat, rye, sunflower seeds, wheat (durum, hard red, hard white), navy beans, pinto beans, mung beans, legumes (Legumes are plants that bare their fruits in pods. Well-known legumes alfalfa, clover, peas, beans, lentils, lupins, mesquite, carob, kidney beans, pinto beans, black eye peas, garbanzo beans, mung beans, soybeans, peanuts, tamarind, and the woody climbing vine wisteria.)

Vitamin B5 (Pantothenic Acid)

Vitamin B5 is essential for growth and metabolism of food and the formulation of hormones as well as (good) cholesterol.

Vitamin B5 Food Source: Avocado, black currants, dates, gooseberries, grapefruit, guava, pomegranate, raspberries, starfruit watermelon, broccoli, brussel sprouts, butternut squash, French beans, mushrooms, okra, pumpkin, spirulina, spaghetti squash, winter squash, whole grain cereals, legumes, white and sweet potatoes, buckwheat, black-eyed peas, soybeans (edamame), lima beans, mung beans, split peas, chestnuts, oats, rye, sunflower seeds, and wheat (durum, hard red, hard white).

Vitamin B6 (Pyridoxine, Pyridoxal, Pyridoxine, Pyridoxamine)

Vitamin B6 is important for protein metabolism, formation of red blood cells and fat usage by your body. Vitamin B6 offers additional support in terms of increased fertility because it balances out the hormone levels. Vitamin B6 focuses mainly on correcting low progesterone levels of women affected by luteal phase defect, in which their luteal phases are not long enough to sustain a successful pregnancy. A normal progesterone level is essential to keep up the pregnancy otherwise it could lead to a miscarriage.

Vitamin B6 Food Source: Banana, bok choy, brussel sprouts, butternut squash, gooseberries, grapes, guava, lychee, mango, passion fruit, pineapple, pomegranate, french beans, green pepper, watermelon, sweet potatoes, kale, lima beans, peas, spirulina, dried prunes, raisins, banana, spaghetti squash, winter squash, chestnuts, hazelnuts, pistachios, pumpkin seeds, sunflower seeds, walnuts, rye, okra, legumes, spinach, avocado, peanut butter, and wheat (durum, hard red, hard white).

Vitamin B7 (Biotin/Vitamin H)

Vitamin B7 is essential for growth and metabolism. It is known that the thyroid and adrenal glands, the nervous system, the reproductive system, and our skin depend on an sufficient supply of this vitamin, Biotin plays a crucial role in metabolizing fats, proteins, and carbohydrates, and several other enzymes involved in the body's metabolic process. It also synthesizes fatty acids, amino acids, keeps blood glucose levels in check, supplements calcium deposits in your nails and keeps them strong, brittle-free.

Vitamin B7 Food Source: Green peas, broccoli, cabbage, cauliflower, sweet potatoes, green and leafy vegetables like spinach, bananas, avocados, strawberries, raspberries, watermelon, grapefruit, oats, soybeans, wheat germ, mushrooms, lentils, split peas, bran, and unpolished brown rice, almonds, pecan, peanuts and walnuts, and brewer's yeast.

Vitamin B9 (Folate/Folic Acid)

Folic acid is an essential vitamin both during pre-conception and pregnancy, as it can prevent spina-bifida in your baby, and other birth defects associated with the brain and spine development in the baby. It used in our bodies to make new cells and helps control blood levels. Also, it is used for protein metabolism, produce DNA, and grow tissues. **In addition, this vitamin promotes sustainable fertility in women and prepares their bodies for pregnancy.** Supplementation with this vitamin

MARLO Y. ETTIEN

is beneficial, since only 50% of the folic acid found in the ingested food can be properly absorbed by the human body.

Vitamin B9 Food Source: Spinach, avocado, blackberries, boysenberries, guava, artichoke, bok choy, buckwheat, chestnuts, rye, quinoa, hazelnuts, peanuts, broccoli, beets, asparagus, beans, legumes, citrus fruits, whole grains, dark green leafy vegetables, mango, loganberries, orange, papaya, pineapple, spirulina, pomegranate, passion fruit, raspberries, soy beans (edamame) strawberries, lima beans, parsnip, romaine lettuce, turnip greens, wheat (durum, hard red, hard white), and sweet potatoes.

Vitamin B12 (Cobalamin)

Vitamin 12 is essential for development of red blood cells, maintenance of nervous system, and metabolism. Deficiency can cause anemia and neurological disorders. **A key vitamin for improved fertility.** Vitamin B12 enhances the occurrence of ovulation, being particularly helpful to women not ovulating at all, making it harder to try to conceive. Vitamin B12 also improves the inner lining of the uterus, thus creating a favorable environment for the implantation of the fertilized eggs. For men, increases sperm motility and sperm count and helps to increase and boost natural *testosterone* production. It also may help to boost the endometrium lining in egg fertilization, decreasing the chances of miscarriage. Some studies have found that a deficiency of B12 may increase the chances of irregular ovulation, and in severe cases stop ovulation altogether.

Vitamin B12 Food Source: Spirulina, chlorella, blue-green algae, brewer's yeast, fortified soy milk, fortified cereals, and B12 supplements.

Vitamin C (Ascorbic Acid)

This excellent antioxidant also aids in both male and female fertility, given the key part it plays in conception. For men, it helps in keeping sperm from clumping together, counteracts the damaging effects of free radicals on the quality of the sperm, and increasing their motility. Also, vitamin helps men maintain healthy testosterone. For women, vitamin C sustains an appropriate female endocrine equilibrium and increases fertility in particular in the case of women having low progesterone levels. It also reinforces the right balance between estrogen and progesterone levels. It will assist with headaches and migraines associated with menopause; and help regulate heavy periods, when combined with bioflavonoids. Vitamin C helps to prevent anemia. During your period, you lose iron as a result of menstrual blood loss. If your

158

period is especially heavy or you have a shorter cycle, you may be at risk for developing iron-deficient anemia, characterized by fatigue and weakness. However, vitamin C allows your body to absorb iron more efficiently, potentially warding off anemia. Clinical trials on women have proven that the chances of getting pregnant doubled following the vitamin C treatment.

Vitamin C Food Source: Oranges, black currants, grapefruit, guava, kiwi, lychee, mango, mulberries, orange, papaya, passion fruit, pineapple, bok choy, brussel sprouts, butternut squash, chestnuts, lemons, limes, clementine, grapefruit, turnip greens, swiss chard, spinach, gold kiwi, broccoli, cranberries, red, yellow, and green peppers, green peas, strawberries, raspberries, blackberries, blueberries, cantaloupe, sweet and white potatoes, and tomatoes.

Vitamin D (calciferol)

Vitamin D is essential to both male and female fertility. It stimulates the levels of estrogen and progesterone, regulates menstruation, and improves the viability of sperm, therefore enhancing a successful outcome. Vitamin D helps your body absorb and regulate calcium and phosphorus in the blood; a mineral which may have a protective role against PMS. In addition, vitamin D may help to regulate hormones and help your neurotransmitters, which affect your mood, to function regularly. A study discussed in the July 2010 issue of "The Journal of Steroid Biochemistry and Molecular Biology" examined vitamin D intake among college-aged women and found that women with a high intake of vitamin D from food sources were less likely to have PMS. In addition, Vitamin D is an essential vitamin during pregnancy with studies showing its use vastly decreasing the risk of preterm labor as well as the risk of other pregnancy complications. Vitamin D is needed to help the body create sex hormones which in turn affects ovulation and hormonal balance.

Vitamin D Food Source: Exposure to sunshine, supplements, and mushrooms (crimini, portabella, shitake, oyster.)

Vitamin E (tocopherol; antioxidant)

Vitamin E is the vitamin of choice for the overall male and female reproductive system. For women, the fertility-friendly vitamin E improves the quality of cervical mucus, thus enhancing the chances of implantation of the fertilized eggs. And moreover, it prolongs the sperm's life within the female a couple more days, so as to increase the chances for the egg to be fertilized. Vitamin E will help with lumpy and tender breasts and assist with headaches and migraines associated with menopause. If you suffer from cramps, vitamin E may provide you with some relief. According to MedlinePlus, vitamin E appears to decrease the duration and severity of cramps, and may even reduce menstrual blood loss. If you also struggle with menstrual migraines too, vitamin E may have additional benefits. A study published in the January 2009 issue of "Medical Science Monitor" found that vitamin E relieved nausea, light sensitivity and sound sensitivity associated with menstrual migraines. Vitamin E helps to improve the overall health of sperm. Sperm can be damaged by harmful molecules (free radicals). Vitamin E is an antioxidant which helps to reduce the number of free radicals. For men, a daily intake of vitamin E is recommended in order to enhance sperm motility.

Vitamin E Food Source: Spinach, asparagus, avocado, orange, mango, papaya, guava, kiwi, nectarine, peach, pomegranate, raspberries, mulberries, tofu, pistachios, turnip greens, collards, kale, cranberries, blueberries, boysenberries, blackberries, black currants, broccoli, butternut squash, potatoes, parsnip, swiss chard, spirulina, green leafy vegetables, almonds, hazelnuts, pine nuts, walnuts, pecans, sunflower seeds, soybeans (edamame) pinto beans, cauliflower, parsley, and banana.

Vitamin K (menaquinone)

Vitamin K is essential for blood clotting and deficiency can cause excessive bleeding. Deficiencies are common in infants or in people who take antibiotics or anticoagulants.

Vitamin K Food Source: Collards, cress, spinach, turnip greens, mustard greens, beet greens, swiss chard, scallions, cauliflower, cress, radiacchio, brussel sprouts, lettuce, broccoli, cabbage, prunes, pear, plum, raspberries, tomatoes, pomegranate, mulberries, grapes, kiwi, loganberries, avocado, blackberries, blueberries, cranberries, boysenberries, prunes, alfalfa sprouted, artichoke, asparagus, cucumber, kale, leeks, okra, peas, cauliflower, celery, cashews, chestnuts, hazelnuts, pine nuts, pistachio, rye, soy beans (edamame), kidney beans, and split peas.

ELECTROLYTES

"**Electrolyte** is a "medical/scientific" term for salts, specifically ions. Electrolytes are salts in the body that conduct electricity and are found in the tissue, and body fluids. For example, your body fluids – blood, plasma, interstitial fluid (fluid between cells) – are like seawater and have a high concentration of **sodium chloride** (table salt, or NaCl). The term electrolyte means that this ion is electrically charged and moves to either a **negative (cathode)** or **positive (anode) electrode**:

- ions that move to the cathode (**cations**) are positively charged.
- ions that move to the anode (**anions**) are negatively charged.

For instance, the electrolytes in sodium chloride (NaCl) are:

- **sodium ion** ($Na+$) - cation
- **chloride ion** ($Cl-$) – anion

Sodium ($Na+$) is concentrated in the extracellular fluid between tissue cells and potassium ($K+$) is concentrated in the intracellular fluid within the blood vessels. Proper balance is essential for muscle coordination, heart function, fluid absorption and excretion, nerve function, and concentration.

As for your body, the major electrolytes are as follows:

1. sodium ($Na+$)
2. potassium ($K+$) 3. chloride ($Cl-$)
4. calcium ($Ca2+$)
5. magnesium ($Mg2+$)
6. bicarbonate ($HCO3-$)
7. phosphate ($PO42-$)
8. sulfate ($SO42-$)

Electrolytes are important because they are what your cells (especially nerve, heart, muscle) use to maintain voltages across their cell membranes and to carry electrical impulses (nerve impulses, muscle contractions) across themselves and to other cells. Your kidneys work to keep the electrolyte concentrations in your blood constant despite changes in your body. For example, when you exercise heavily, you lose electrolytes in your sweat, particularly sodium and potassium. These electrolytes must be replaced to keep the electrolyte concentrations of your body fluids constant."

MINERALS

"BORON (B) – Trace Mineral
Builds strong healthy bones and muscles as well as helps prevent bone loss. It aids in improving the thinking function.

Boron Food Source: Leafy green vegetables, legumes, red apples, carrots, grapes, nuts, pears, whole grains, raisins, prunes, peanuts, honey, broccoli, bananas, chick peas, onions, oranges, walnuts, almonds, avocados, pears, green beans, hazelnuts, dandelion, parsley, pig weed, cabbage, and garlic.

CALCIUM (Ca) – Major Mineral
Insufficient calcium in the body can affect the bones which may lead to osteoporosis, high blood pressure and colon cancer. Another effect involves sensations of numbness and tingling around the mouth and fingertips and painful aches and spasms of the muscles. Getting enough calcium can ease the symptoms of premenstrual syndrome (PMS). An adequate supply of calcium helps muscles, including your heart muscle, do their work of contracting and relaxing. Calcium also appears to help regulate pressure in arteries to nervous system.

Calcium Food Source: Blackberries, blackcurrants, grapes, dates, mulberries, orange, pomegranates, prickly pears, amaranth leaves, bok choy, brussel sprouts, butternut squash, celery, Chinese broccoli, french beans, kale, okra, parsnip, spirulina, swiss chard, turnip, brazil nuts, almond, oats, pistachios, sesame seeds, wheat (duram and hard) soy beans (edamame), white beans, winged beans, navy beans, asparagus, barley, basil, zucchini, lemon, tangerine, mustard, greens, thyme, hummus, eggplant, black beans, lentils, tofu, parsley, lima beans, pinto beans, garlic, coriander, winter squash, figs, apricots, prunes, watercress, cabbage, kelp, spinach, and tempeh.

CHLORIDE (Cl) – Trace Mineral Two types: Sodium and Calcium
When too much salt in the body increases, the combined phenomena of low blood pressure and feeling of weakness are symptoms of a chloride deficiency. When this chloride mineral drops down, the body experience loss of potassium via the urine. This is a dangerous condition that causes the blood pH level to become elevated. Affected person can lose the ability to control muscle function leading to problems with breathing, swallowing and even death.

Chloride Food Sources: Kelp, and tomatoes.

CHROMIUM (Cr) – Trace Mineral

Participates in assisting our body to absorb and stabilize energy that we need throughout the day. Sufficient quantity of it can make many large biological molecules that help us survive. It can also help increase muscle mass while reducing fat mass in our bodies. But it is often difficult to get enough chromium in our diets. People who exercise frequently have especially high demands for this element.

Chromium Food Source: Broccoli, brewer's yeast, whole wheat, rye, tomato, spinach, sweet potatoes with skin, dried beans, onion, garlic, barley, oats, green beans, romaine lettuce, wild yam, nettle, catnip, oat straw, licorice, horsetail, yarrow, red clover and sarsaparilla, and brown rice.

COBALT (Co) – Trace Mineral

Without cobalt, Vitamin B-12 could not exist. The body uses this vitamin for numerous of purposes like digestion and nerve function where B12 deficiency can also cause nerve cells to form incorrectly, resulting in irreversible nerve damage. This situation is characterized by symptoms such as delusions, eye disorders, dizziness, confusion, and memory loss. B-12 is necessary for the normal formation of all cells, especially red blood cells. Strict vegetarians are at risk of B-12 deficiency because vegetables do not contain this important vitamin. B-12 can be found nutritional yeast, and in animal sources such as red meat, fish, eggs, cheese, and milk. Alternatively, you can get plenty of vitamin B-12 from most multi-vitamin supplements.

Cobalt Food Sources: Green leafy vegetables as spinach and kale, nuts, oat cereals, cayenne pepper, dandelion, and echinacea.

COPPER (Cu) – Trace Mineral

Is a necessary part of the body's ability to produce hemoglobin. It also works together with iron in the formation of red blood cells. Without copper, the body could not complete the process of building the bones that make up the skeletal system. When the body experiences this rare deficiency, it also means a deficiency in iron. Symptoms like anemia, anorexia nervosa, starvation and kidney problems are taken account from this.

Copper Food Source: Avocado, kiwi, blackberries, dates, guava, lychee, mango, passionfruit, pomegranate, amaranth leaves, artichoke, french beans, kale, lima beans, parsnip, peas, potatoes, pumpkin, spirulina, winter squash, celery, garlic, radishes, mushrooms, pecans, cocoa, prunes, bananas, cherries, raisins, barley, artichokes, sweet potatoes, swiss chard, taro, brazil nuts, buckwheat, cashews, chestnuts, filberts/hazelnuts, oats, sunflower seeds, walnuts, Wheat/durum and hard red, adzuki beans, kidney beans, white beans, dried prunes, black beans, black eye peas, fava beans soy beans/ edamame, lima beans, navy beans, pigeon beans, pinto beans, and winged beans.

GERANIUM (GE) – Trace Mineral

Helps in healthy functioning of the immune system and aids the body in cleansing toxins and wound healing. It also helps to fight pain. One of its main functions is to stimulate cells to increase their intake of oxygen and provide the body more energy.

Geranium Food Sources: Wheat, bran, legumes, tomato juice, broccoli, celery, garlic, onions, shitake mushrooms, rhubarb, sauerkraut, aloe vera, comfrey chlorella, and ginseng.

IODINE (I) – Trace Mineral

Seventy-five percent of this mineral makes its way to the thyroid gland then joins up with two important hormones - triiodothyronine and thyroxin. Every part of the body requires these hormones to produce energy. These hormones determine how fast and how efficiently the body is able to burn calories. This can make the amount of fat in the blood supply to increase, thyroid gland can become enlarged, and hoarseness can develop in the throat and in children, may cause mental retardation.

Iodine Food Sources: Kelp, navy beans, cranberries, iodized salt, strawberries, kombu, and potatoes.

IRON (Fe) Trace Mineral

It is easy to get enough iron if we can be able to maintain a balance diet. But ironically, iron deficiency anemia is the most common nutritional disease in the world affecting at least five million people to this date. Iron is crucial element to sustain healthy immune system, digestion, and hemoglobin which is carrier of oxygen to our body. In addition, certain chemicals in our brain are controlled by the presence or absence of iron. Studies have shown that women who do not get sufficient amounts of iron may suffer anovulation (lack of ovulation) and possibly poor egg health, which can inhibit pregnancy at a rate 60% higher than those with sufficient iron stores in their blood.

Iron Food Source: Blackberries, avocado, boysenberries, blackcurrant, breadfruits, cherries, dates, figs grapes, kiwi, lemon, loganberries, lychee, mulberries, passion fruit, persimmon, pomegranate, raspberry, strawberry, watermelon, peas, potatoes, pumpkin seeds, amaranth leave, bok choy, brussel sprout, leeks, kale, swiss chard, spirulina, lima beans, french beans, butternut squash, coconut, pine nuts, wheat (duram and hard), spelts, rye, cashews, adzumi beans, black beans, pinto beans, white beans, navy beans, navy beans, pigeon peas, split peas, winged beans, mung beans, kidney beans, garbanzo beans, black eye peas, blueberries, strawberries, bananas, mango, garlic, tomatoes, celery, burdock, Echinacea, yarrow, chickweed, red clover, sunflower seeds, pumpkin seeds, molasses, cashews, peanuts, and paprika.

MAGNESIUM (Mg) – Major Mineral

Amazingly plays an important role in about 300 biochemical processes that take place inside the body. This is needed to properly develop and maintain the skeletal system and very crucial to body's ability to absorb calcium. Magnesium deficiency can lead a person to experience heart disease, diabetes and osteoporosis. It also reveals that it can help to keep muscles and mind relaxed. Migraine, numbness, muscle cramps, anxiety problem and changes in personality can be symptoms in lacking sufficient magnesium.

Magnesium Food Source: Lemon, zucchini, tangerine, nectarines, artichokes, plums, whole wheat bread, coconut milk, cranberries, apricots, honeydew, papaya, prunes, cauliflower, garlic, asparagus, barley, basil, peppers, pepper, brussel sprouts, buckwheat, cashews, chili peppers, coriander, dill, fennel, figs, flaxseed, onions, hazelnuts, leeks, lima beans, millet, shiitake mushrooms, rosemary, mustard greens, navy beans, parsley, pinto beans, rye, sesame seeds, soy sauce, soy beans, summer squash, winter squash, sunflower seeds, swiss chard, thyme, tempeh, turnip greens, a shake, chocolate, chia seeds, spirulina, quinoa, watermelon, dates, guava, lima beans, avocado, blackberries, raspberries, pinto beans, okra, oats, peanuts, cantaloupe, peach, pineapple, grapefruit, mango, dill, basil, rosemary, spearmint, and peppermint.

MANGANESE (Mn) – Trace Mineral

Manganese is not only antioxidant but also responsible in developing bones, metabolic process, and reproduction function. A manganese deficiency can cause painful joints, osteoporosis, memory loss and diabetes.

Manganese Food Source: Blackberries, blueberries, raspberries, avocado, blackcurrant, guava, grapefruit, gooseberries, loganberries, pineapples, pomegranate, strawberries, dates, cranberries, boysenberries, peas, potatoes, spirulina, kale, leeks, lima beans, parsnip, butternut squash, sweet potato, swiss chard, buckwheat, coconut, pecans, macadamia nuts, pine nuts, almonds, hazelnuts, grapes, kiwi, garlic, mustard greens, cloves, turmeric, leeks, cucumber, peppermint, coconuts, bananas, molasses, beet root, watercress, lettuce, blackberries, soy beans, white beans, winged beans, pigeon beans, garbanzo beans, potatoes, brussel sprouts, french beans, taro, brazil nuts, cashews, amaranth leaves, black tea, saffron, and ginger.

MOLYBDENUM (Mo) – Trace Mineral

Is important in helping our cells grow. Small amount of molybdenum promotes healthy teeth and rand gum problems, lack of oxygen in the blood, loss of appetite and weight.

Molybdenum Food Sources: Navy beans, lentils, black eye peas, split peas, lima beans, kidney beans, almonds, chestnuts, peanuts, cashews, soybeans, black beans, chick peas, green leafy vegetables, seeds, green beans, and tomatoes.

NICKEL (Ni)—Trace Mineral

It helps activate certain enzymes and involved in the activity of hormones and cell membrane. Low blood levels of Nickel are observed in people with vitamin B6 deficiency, cirrhosis of the liver, and kidney failure. Elevated blood levels of nickel, on the other hand, are associated with the development of cancer, heart attack, thyroid disorders, psoriasis and eczema. This suggests the need of balance intake to avoid the opposite negative results.

Nickel Food Source: Cocoa, cashews, kidney beans, spinach, dried apricot, figs, and prunes, soy beans (edamame), chick peas/garbanzo beans, lentils, yellow peas, mung beans, peanuts, hazelnuts, almonds, walnuts, oat bran, buckwheat, wheat, and millet.

PHOSPHORUS (P) – Major Mineral

Phosphorus helps with maintaining healthy blood sugar levels. Phosphorus is also found in substantial amounts in the nervous system. Phosphorus deficiency can occur among people who take certain types of antacids for longer years. People who become easily fatigued and weak can be symptoms of mild phosphate deficiency. However, too much intake of it through taking processed foods, soft drinks and meats may lead to osteoporosis.

Phosphorus Food Source: Bananas, apples, oranges, watermelon, strawberries, avocado, blueberries, broccoli, almonds, cucumber, honey, pears, pineapple, cantaloupe, celery, oatmeal, cherries, grapefruit, brown rice, tomatoes, mushrooms, potatoes, salad, sweet potato, green beans, butternut squash, peanuts, pumpkin seeds, quinoa, a mango, mango, pecans, raisins, spinach, spirulina, walnuts, oats, cabbage, beets, garbanzo beans, tofu, kiwi, lentils, pomegranate, kale, black beans, coconut, dates, kidney beans, hummus, eggplant, lemon, zucchini, tangerine, nectarines, artichokes, plums, cranberries, apricots, honeydew, papaya, prunes, prune juice, cauliflower, garlic, brazil nuts, sunflower seeds, spelt, rye, pine nuts, black eye peas, kidney beans, lima beans, pinto beans, garbanzo beans, navy beans, white beans, and parsley.

POTASSIUM (K) – Major Mineral

We should have balance intake of Sodium to avoid heart disease and benefit from maintaining balance of positive and negative ions in our body fluids and tissues. Sodium aids in preventing heat prostration or sunstroke. Deficient of sodium can reduce body water and sodium to the extent that gross dehydration affects normal activity patterns.

Potassium: Avocado, blackcurrants, bananas, breadfruit, cherimoya, cherries, Chinese pear, grapefruit, dates, guava, kiwi, lychee, papaya, passion fruit, pomegranate, prickly pear, watermelon, swiss chard, sweet potatoes, garlic, spirulina, pumpkin, parsnip, lima beans, French beans, butternut squash, bok choy, bamboo shoots, amaranth leaves, almonds, buckwheat, chestnuts, coconut, oats, pistachios, pumpkin seeds, sunflower seeds, rye, wheat (durum, hard), adzuki beans, pinto beans, lima beans, soy beans, white beans, kidney beans, swiss chard, kale, zucchini, spinach, mushroom, Brussel sprouts, green beans, asparagus, thyme, parsley, basil, black beans, lemons, cabbage, beets, mustard greens, cashews, hazelnuts, cucumber, and turnip greens.

SELENIUM (Se) – Trace Mineral

Is cancer-fighting potential, which has antioxidant properties. This means it protects against the formation of free radicals - unstable oxygen molecules in the body caused by muscle movement, metabolism and inhalation of smoke and pollution. An antioxidant that helps to protect the eggs and sperm from free radicals. Free radicals can cause chromosomal damage which is known to be a cause of miscarriages and birth defects. Selenium is also necessary for the creation of sperm. In studies men with low sperm counts have also been found to have low levels of selenium.

Selenium Food Source: Brazil nuts, bananas, breadfruit, guava, lychee, mango, passion fruit, pomegranate, watermelon, lima beans, peas, parsnip, mushrooms (shitake, crimini and button), spirulina, French beans, asparagus, Brussel sprouts, mung beans, navy beans, pigeon beans, plantains, spinach, black eye peas, fava beans, wheat, barley, brown rice, oats, garlic, ginger, parsley, garlic, onions, lentils, brown rice, brazil nuts, broccoli, grapefruit, and amaranth.

SILICON (Si) – Major Mineral

This element is important in the functioning of nerve cells and tissues because it controls the transmission of nerve impulses. It is also called 'beauty mineral,' because it protects the eyes and skin and essential for the growth of our teeth, nails, and hair. For diseases like tuberculosis, irritations in the mucous membranes and skin disorders - silicon contributes for the healing processes.

Silicon Food Source: Romaine lettuce, almonds, flaxseeds, millet, almonds, peanuts, tomato, nopal cactus, radish, spinach, marjoram, horsetail, hemp leaves, cucumber, grapes, raisins, oranges, apples, burdock root, barley, beets, brown rice, oats, soy beans, bell peppers, bananas, whole wheat, and alfalfa, blue cohosh, comfrey, leafy green vegetables, chickweed, dandelion, red raspberry, stinging nettles, red peppers, celery, beets, potatoes, carrots, cornsilk, and red lentils.

SODIUM (Na) – Major Mineral

Sodium is important in the distribution of water in the body. It helps in maintenance of fluid volume in the vessels and tissues and also concerned with muscle and nerve irritability.

Sodium Food Source: Guava, strawberry, passion fruit, amaranth leaves, coconut, winged beans, artichoke, beetroot, broccoli, bok choy, Brussel sprouts, celery, fennel, kale, spirulina, spaghetti squash, sweet potato, swiss chard, pumpkin seeds, quinoa, spelt, winged beans, tamarinds, honeydew, cantaloupe, mulberries, kumquats, and strawberries.

SULFUR (S) – Major Mineral

This essential element can easily be found in all food that we eat so we don't have to get worried about. Sulfur defends the body cells from environmental hazards such as air pollution and radiation. In addition, sulfur helps our liver function correctly, helps us digest the food that we eat and then turn that food into energy. Remarkable discovery found that it can help in the aging process to slow down and extends our life span. It keeps our skin supple and elastic as well. If you get sulfur more than your body needs, you just excrete it in your urine.

Sulfur Food Source: garlic, lettuce, cabbage, brussel sprouts, broccoli, cauliflower, cabbage, kale, turnips, bok choy, and kohlrabi, walnuts, almonds, sesame seeds, sunflower seeds, coconut, banana, watermelon, mustard greens, water cress, kale, garlic, onions, dried beans, asparagus, leeks, peas, chives, avocado, peanuts, pistachios, and wheat germ.

TIN (Sn) – Trace Mineral

Primarily supports the function of the adrenal gland. Psychological benefits include decreased depression and fatigue, an increase in positive mood and general well-being, and an increase in energy. Some test subjects also experienced improvements in general occurrences of pain, skin problems, and digestion. There was also a noticeable decrease in headaches, asthma, and insomnia for some.

Tin Food Source: Kelp, figs, dog grass, juniper, bilberry, milk thistle, dulse, lady slipper, althea, valerian, Irish moss, nettle, barberry, yarrow, blessed thistle, yellow dock, licorice, devils claw, pennyroyal, and senna. Found in all fruits and vegetables.

VANADIUM (V) – Trace Mineral

There might also be some potential health benefits provided by vanadium for those with bipolar disorder. Researchers believe that when people are in the manic state of bipolar disorder their vanadium levels are significantly elevated, which means that a diet which reduces vanadium intake may actually be beneficial to those with bipolar disorder.

Vanadium Food Source: Mushrooms, parsley, dill weed, buckwheat, green beans, corn, carrots, radishes, oats, cabbage, garlic, tomatoes, onions, olives, snap beans, black pepper.

ZINC (Zn) – Trace Mineral

Sixty-seven percent of US population suffers from zinc deficiency. Sufficient requirement of this can ensure that the immune system remains healthy and is able to fight off disease. It helps produce and activate T-lymphocytes, one type of white blood cell that the body uses to help fight infection. It can hamper sexual function and capability, impotence, lethargy, loss of appetite and diminished immune capability. In women, zinc works with more than three hundred different enzymes in the body to keep things working well.

Without it, your cells can not divide properly; your estrogen and progesterone levels can get out of balance and your reproductive system may not be fully functioning. Low levels of zinc have been linked to miscarriage in the initial stages of a pregnancy, according to The Centers for Disease Control's Assisted Reproductive Technology Report.

In men zinc is considered one of the most important trace minerals to date for male fertility; increasing zinc levels in infertile men has been shown to boost sperm levels; improve the form, function and quality of male sperm and decrease male infertility.

Zinc Food Source: Bananas, apples, oranges, wine, watermelon, strawberry, avocado, blueberries, broccoli, almonds, cucumber, pears, pineapple, cantaloupe, peaches, celery, cherries, grapefruit, brown rice, tomatoes, mushrooms, potatoes, sweet potato, nuts, orange juice, green beans, tuna, skim milk, fish, butternut squash, peanuts, pumpkin seeds, quinoa, mango, pecans, raisins, spinach, spirulina, walnuts, oats, cabbage, beets, garbanzo beans, tofu, kiwi, lentils, pomegranate, kale, black beans, coconut, dates, kidney beans, hummus, eggplant, lemon, zucchini, tangerine, nectarines, artichokes, plums, cranberries, apricots, honeydew, papaya, prunes, cauliflower, garlic, asparagus, barley, basil, brussel sprouts, buckwheat, cashews, chili peppers, coriander, dill, fennel, figs, flaxseed, tea, onions, yams, hazelnuts, leeks, lima beans, millet, shiitake mushrooms, rosemary, mustard greens, navy beans, parsley, pinto beans, rye, sesame seeds, soy beans, summer squash, winter squash, sunflower seeds, swiss chard, thyme, tempeh, turnip greens, chia seeds, brewer's yeast, and pecans."

AMINO ACIDS (INCLUDING 3-LETTER AND 1-LETTER IDENTIFIERS)

1. Alanine (Ala) (A) – Nonessential
2. Arginine (Arg) (R) – Nonessential
3. Asparagine (Asn) (N) — Nonessential
4. Aspartic acid (Asp) (D) — Nonessential
5. Cysteine (Cys) (C) – Nonessential
6. Cystine (Cys) (C) — Nonessential
7. Glutamine (Gln) (Q) – Nonessential
8. Glutamic acid (Glu) (E) — Nonessential
9. Glycine (Gly) (G) — Nonessential
10. Histidine (His) (H) – Nonessential
11. Hydroxyproline (Hyp) (H) – Nonessential
12. Isoleucine (Ile) (I) — Essential
13. Leucine (Leu) (L) — Essential
14. Lysine (Lys) (K) — Essential
15. Methionine (Met) (M) — Essential
16. Phenylalanine (Phe) (F) — Essential
17. Proline (Pro) (P) — Nonessential
18. Serine (Ser) (S) — Nonessential
19. Threonine (Thr) (T) — Essential
20. Tryptophan (Trp) (W) — Essential
21. Tyrosine (Tyr) (Y) — Nonessential
22. Valine (Val) (V) — Essential

ALANINE (Non-Essential Amino Acid)

Is an important source of energy for muscle tissue, the brain and central nervous system; strengthens the immune system by producing antibodies; helps in the metabolism of sugars and organic acids.

ARGININE (Non-Essential Amino Acid)

It improves immune responses to bacteria, viruses & tumor cells; promotes wound healing and regeneration of the liver; causes the release of growth hormones; considered crucial for optimal muscle growth and tissue repair. Arginine stimulates the growth of new bone and tendon cells.

ASPARAGINE (Non-Essential Amino Acid)

On intracellular function, Asparagine, Glutamine and Serine are vital for energy and smooth function of brain reactions; contribute to the formation of proteins, muscles, neurotransmitters, ,antibodies and receptors. Asparagine is an important transporters of nitrogen; foundation of carbohydrate metabolism; improves recovery after surgery or trauma by hastening wound.

ASPARTIC ACID (Non-Essential Amino Acid)

Aspartic Acid aids in the expulsion of harmful ammonia from the body. When ammonia enters the Circulatory System, it acts as a highly toxic substance which can be harmful to the Central Nervous System.

CYSTEINE (Non-Essential Amino Acid)

In addition to protecting the cells from the harmful effects of radiation, [L-Cysteine] protects the liver and brain from damage due to alcohol and cigarette smoke. It functions as an antioxidant and is a powerful aid to the body in protecting against radiation and pollution. It can help slow down the aging process, deactivate free radicals, neutralize toxins; and aids in protein synthesis and presents cellular change. It is necessary for the formation of the skin, which aids in the recovery from burns and surgical operations. Hair and skin are made up 10-14% Cystine.

GLUTAMINE (Non-Essential Amino Acid)

The brain requires a constant supply of energy to think and be alert, Glutamine provides the fuel the brain cells need to think clearly and help combat fatigue.

GLUTAMIC ACID (Non-Essential Amino Acid)

Considered to be nature's "Brain food" by improving mental capacities; helps speed the healing of ulcers; support your digestive track; gives a "lift" from fatigue; helps control alcoholism, schizophrenia, and the craving for sugar.

GLYCINE (Non-Essential Amino Acid)

Helps trigger the release of oxygen to the energy requiring cell-making process; Important in the manufacturing of hormones responsible for a strong immune system.

HISTIDINE (Non-Essential Amino Acid)

Is found abundantly in hemoglobin; has been used in the treatment of rheumatoid arthritis, allergic diseases, ulcers & anemia. A deficiency can cause poor hearing.

HYDROXYPROLINE (Non-Essential Amino Acid)
Plays a major role in manufacture of collagen, connective tissue, skin, ligaments, tendons, bones, cartilage and is necessary in Vitamin D assimilation. Vitamin D is essential in proper calcium absorption.

ISOLEUCINE (Essential Amino Acid)
Isoleucine stimulates the brain to produce alertness.

LEUCINE (Essential Amino Acid)
Leucine stimulates protein synthesis and its importance in protein storage. Both Isoleucine and Leucine provide ingredients for the manufacturing of other essential biochemical components in the body, some of which are utilized for the production of energy—stimulants to the upper brain and helping you to be more alert.

LYSINE (Essential Amino Acid)
Lysine is found in the muscle tissue. Soybeans are high in lysine, but rare in other vegetables. Lysine ensures the adequate absorption of calcium; helps form collagen (which makes up bone cartilage & connective tissues); aids in the production of antibodies, hormones & enzymes. A deficiency may result in tiredness, inability to concentrate, irritability, bloodshot eyes, retarded growth, hair loss, anemia & reproductive problems.

METHIONINE (Essential Amino Acid)
Methionine performs the major roles of being a methyl donor, sulfur donor, and helps lower cholesterol. Methionine is a natural chelating agent for heavy metals; is a principle supplier of sulfur which prevents disorders of the hair, skin and nails; influences hair follicles and promotes hair growth; increases the liver's production of lecithin thus helps reduce cholesterol and liver fat; regulates the formation of ammonia and creates ammonia-free urine which reduces bladder irritation and promotes kidney health.

PHENYLALAINE (Essential Amino Acid)
Phenylamine, which is highly concentrated in protein foods is understood to perform as a pain reliever. Phenylalanine is used by the brain to produce norepinephrine, a chemical that transmits signals between nerve cells and the brain. It helps maintain alertness; reduces hunger; acts as an antidepressant and helps improve memory.

PROLINE (Non-Essential Amino Acid)
Essential for proper functioning of joints and tendons; helps maintain and strengthen heart muscles.

SERINE (Non-Essential Amino Acid)
Is a storage source of glucose by the liver and muscles; helps strengthen the immune system by providing antibodies; synthesizes fatty acid sheath around nerve fibers.

THREONINE (Essential Amino Acid)
Threonine is the least abundant amino acid, but essential in preventing fat build-up in the liver and assisting digestive and intestinal tracts function more smoothly; assists metabolism and assimilation. Threonine is an important constituent of collagen, Elastin, and enamel protein.

TRYPTOPHAN (Essential Amino Acid)
Tryptophan is a natural relaxant, helps alleviate insomnia by inducing normal sleep; reduces anxiety & depression; helps in the treatment of migraine headaches; helps the immune system controlling certain intractable pain; helps reduce the risk of artery & heart spasms; works with Lysine in reducing cholesterol levels.

TYROSINE (Non-Essential Amino Acid)
Transmits nerve impulses to the brain; helps overcome depression; Improves memory; increases mental alertness; and promotes the healthy functioning of the thyroid, adrenal and pituitary glands. Tyrosine is synthesized in the body from phenylalanine. Like phenylalanine, tyrosine is intimately involved with the important brain neurotransmitters epinephrine, norepinephrine, and dopamine.

VALINE (Essential Amino Acid)
Valine promotes mental vigor, muscle coordination and calms emotions.

Appendixes

What is Biofeedback?

"Biofeedback is a non-invasive diagnostic and treatment device based on Quantum Physics widely used by all health care professionals around the World. In the U.S.A. it is registered with the FDA as a class II medical device.

The Bio-feedback device is a technique in which clients are trained to improve their health by using signals from their own bodies electrical system. Biofeedback and Neuro-feedback trains mind and body to make changes in life using a sophisticated medical software program to identify ENERGETIC IMBALANCES & WEAKNESS in the body. Acting like a virus scan on a computer, the EPFX-SCIO system can detect and measure up to twelve thousand deficiencies or imbalances in the human body. One will never know how many of those abnormalities the body has, or if any, until a qualified and knowledgeable Practitioner does a Bio-feedback SCAN. After measuring or scanning the body's electrical frequencies, the system performs THERAPIES to neutralize and BALANCE the destructive energetic pattern that is detected during that session with the client. EPFX-SCIO system can detect a person's internal bodily function with precise sensitivity and precision more than the person themselves can.

The information received can pave the way to a great HEALING of the diseased body. During a Bio-feedback session, the system may add frequency and in others reverse it to either enhance or counteract the body's own resonances, all to rebalance the body to bring relief of ailments and conditions. Clinical Bio-feedback techniques that grew out of the early laboratory procedures are now widely used to treat an ever-lengthening list of conditions. These includes nutritional/allergy testing, migraine headache , tension headaches and many other types of pain, disorders of the digestive system, high or low blood pressure, cardiac arrhythmias (abnormalities in the rhythm of the heartbeat), Raynaud's disease, (a circulatory disorder that causes uncomfortably cold hands), anxiety, depression, bipolar depression, tuning the brain waves, emotional growth, NL , cellular detoxification, addiction release, ADD/ADHD, learning disabilities, behavioral issues, candida, yeast infection, chronic fatigue, fibromyalgia, fungal infection, parasites, pathogens, PMS, memory loss, mental disorders and many more

Bio-feedback therapy can be conducted on the premises or off premises."

APPENDIX B

Promise Ring Gathering Announcement and Story

Announcement e-mail to our circle dated Wednesday, May 19, 2010 @ approximately 10:59 a.m.:

"I hope all is well. Yesterday was Banvoa's one-year anniversary for experiencing her period. It has been a very intimate and nurturing year between us that has simply been amazing. For those of you who participated in the party last year, you will be glad to know that she is using the mugs, has used the lotions and soaps, is reading the books, has drank the teas (green tea, and chamomile with lavender are her favorites). She has used everything from the baskets over the year.

As a follow-up to the Flowering Party, I would like to have a Promise Ring Gathering for Banvoa on Saturday, June 19th. I thought about the next major step in her development as a young girl regarding her body, and this is to discuss sexuality. Typically, young girls receive a promise ring from a boy. The promise ring I am offering to Banvoa symbolizes the promise that she makes with herself regarding her own body.

So, The Promise Ring Gathering is an extension of the Flowering Party. It is an acknowledgement of the importance of Banvoa continuing to embrace the sacredness of her body as well as being another special moment for us to come back together to reflect, share more stories, and gifts. Peace and Blessings. Love, Marlo"

We were all blessed to have the party Saturday, June 19th. As someone who enjoys sharing stories, knowing how encouraging and life giving they are, please enjoy the Promise Ring Gathering story as well:

Promise Ring Gathering Story

Greetings All,

The Promise Ring Gathering was absolutely PHENOMENAL!! It was a tremendous outpouring of love that we are still basking in the glow of. I will soon send pictures. As for details and highlights, the gathering started at 4 p.m.. The only change in the menu below was an apple tart rather than apple turnovers from the bakery. There were ten of us. Linda had a family reunion out of town, and Madina became ill with a virus. Rickenya (Hannah) and Toni (Alex) brought their daughters. After everyone got acquainted, we gathered around the dinner table to bless the food. As we were eating the cake, I reminded everyone, once we finished eating the cake we would have prayer, offer Banvoa the keepsake box, and have woman talk. We gathered in a circle in the family room and had prayer was led by me and anyone who wanted to pray would follow in turn. During my prayer, I invoked the names of the women who were not physically present to complete our circle. What was fascinating about the prayer circle is as every woman prayed the circle got tighter, the bond between us was strengthened. You could feel the presence of the All in the midst of us. When the prayer got around to Rickenya, the power of her prayer grabbed us, connected us on an even deeper level. Whatever needed to fall off, whatever clarity you needed was brought to the fore with her prayer. The power was as lightening striking a tree.

Toni completed the circle in standing next to me. As the prayer went around and led to Toni, she sang "The Lord's Prayer," which was absolutely RIVETING–just riveting, which closed our prayer. Whatever you needed to be cleansed of got cleansed by the end of the song. After we released the circle, I unexpectedly cried. There was so much love shared, I could not hold back my tears. I felt so much security, not just for myself as a mother to have such strong and beautiful women as a part of my circle, I felt security for Banvoa. She is protected and sealed by the strength of our love. I was comforted and assured, and I just held and embraced Banvoa and through my tears, shared with the women that I did not know that I could love a child as much as I love Banvoa. We all know that I can because of Emmanuel. However, for a few years before him, I was not so sure. My love for Banvoa is not compensating for anything that I did not receive from my own mother. It just is. After the prayer, we offered the keepsake box. Banvoa read everything and was overwhelmed by all that she received. Included in the keepsake box was a gift from Armel, Ed Hardy perfume that she wanted and a special note that he wrote, which I read. After we shared everything, I offered her the ring as a promise to keep her body sacred and encouraged her to remain abstinent until she was ready to share her body with her husband through marriage. I told her I expected her to wear the ring until she was thirty. Well, I let go just a little, and said twenty-five. It was such a wonderful time.

Then there was the woman talk and you just had to be there. It was incredible. It was led by the elder in the group, Aunt Gwen, who picked up where she left off a year ago, continuing the discussion about who a virtuous woman is and what she does, which I thought was a wonderful continuation of an unbroken circle—to pick-up where we left off last year at the start of Banvoa entering into womanhood and have the elder lead and guide us with her wisdom. And all of us chimed into what the elder said, sharing our own experiences and lessons we needed to teach Banvoa and Alex (Toni's preteen daughter). After the gathering ended a little after eight, as we were cleaning up, I asked Banvoa what she thought of everything, what was most important to her, and she said Aunt Gwen's advice, her wisdom. I could see Banvoa and Aunt Gwen communicating as she spoke directly to Banvoa, it was an unsaid conversation. We were all bearing witness to the elder's shaping and molding Banvoa's character with her wise words— helping her soul to grow in the way that a good farmer cultivates crops. I could see the intergenerational connectedness of an elder who has lived and seen many things and was honest and open to share with Banvoa what she has learned and observe Banvoa receive it with tenderness and respect by listening intently. It was captivating. There was so much honor being offered, being shared. It was a beautiful experience of healing and newness. There was so much more said, and it was all sacred. Every woman spoke her truth, sharing wisdom. As I have said, every girl should have a Flowering Party and Promise Ring Gathering to help carry them along their life's journey. Although this was our bonding as women, the next morning I took pictures of Armel offering Banvoa the ring. He wanted to share more in our experience because of Banvoa being his daughter and being so close to her. I shared with everyone at the gathering, when talking about boys, how Armel calls the school every day to make sure she made it safely. I learned this last year after the Flowering Party. Well, Banvoa is blooming into our beautiful flower. I feel a great expansion in my life, an inner quiet and peace. Thank you all for sharing. Let us all watch and "see what the end will be."
Love and Blessings,
Marlo

APPENDIX C

Promise Ring Gathering Reflections
Most of the women offered their reflection about the gathering:

The promise ring gathering was a wonderful bonding experience for me. I did not know what to expect as I showed up to Marlo's house with her beautifully draped in African attire as always, stirring potato salad and smiling at me with the most welcoming smile. I was first greeted at the door by the honoree Banvoa, who was

beautiful and corrected me promptly and proudly as I mispronounced her name. It had been a while since I had been to someone's house that was so inviting, so beautiful and so much like home (I work a lot and don't get out much). As I sat and watched Marlo in all of her feminine glory it was amazing to me. Most times I see her in work mode, so it was wonderful just to be with her in sister mode sharing the experience of motherhood/host. Then as all of the women arrived each one with their own style and beauty I was pleased at the natural progression of sisterhood and bonding that took place as the evening went on. I definitely showed up at this event to support Marlo and Banvoa but ended up feeling supported, supportive, and embraced by everyone in the room. It was one of the most powerful gatherings I have been to in a long time. The prayer was most impactful to me as each sister spoke her truth in the presence of the Most High and then that song, the Lord's Prayer, Wow!!!! Just took me out (in a good way!) Yes, this was definitely one for the memory books. Thank you, Marlo, for the love and for being such a supportive and wonderful mother and at the end of the gathering I had to say thank you to Banvoa for bringing us all together, as we all came there to share with her, and I think I can safely say we all got what we needed as well. I look forward to all women everywhere being able to share in this wonderful experience of sisterhood; what a blessing and I was happy to be a part. And to all of you who were in attendance thank you for your wisdom, support, and love. Until we meet again, may love have its way with you......
Love you all Malane

Ephesians 4:16 (Amplified Bible)
For because of Him the whole body (the church, in all its various parts), closely joined and firmly knit together by the joints and ligaments with which it is supplied, when each part [with power adapted to its need] is working properly [in all its functions], grows to full maturity, building itself up in love. It was a privilege to participate and fellowship with a group of women who came together (as one body) to provide guidance to a young lady moving towards womanhood. While the evening started off quietly it was one that was filled with peace and love. Later, as we became acquainted with one another laughter flowed through the room, you could feel the joy of one's voice as they spoke. Then, as we moved toward prayer, the Holy Spirit, the One who Was and Is to come, began to make His everlasting presence known to each person present. It was truly a beautiful experience for us all. I pray this will be a memorial (one that can be reflected upon; one of love) for Banvoa as she moves forward to be the woman that God has called her to be. I am glad that my daughter at the age of five was able to participate, may she also remember this day of prayer and love.
Rickenya

The Promise Ring Gathering was spiritual and provided a great platform to help Banvoa receive wisdom from so many wonderful women who were there. It was a celebration of her development into womanhood because it provided a fantastic opportunity for her to sit at the feet of wisdom, which was expressed through her favorite foods, gifts, songs, prayers. Most of all, it reflected that tender care and love that her mother demonstrated by creating such a ceremonial venue which celebrated Banvoa in such an impressive way. I also loved the fact that Armel, her father, was included in the ceremony by placing the ring on her finger. In our culture, the family has balance because the male and female are integral components of our children's healthy development.
Much Love, Ursula

My experience was quite surprising to me. I just thought I would help serve, eat a little, and dip later on to be about my business! lol But I was overwhelmed with happiness, thankfulness, and a sincere desire to be supportive of my little cousin. I am very proud of you Marlo, and I hope to one day be as good a mother as you are to both your children. I was initially shocked at the whole concept and felt a little uneasy - but now I get it! I even feel a little more comfortable with my own body as I have helped you out on your project. I appreciate the opportunity to speak, and I pray Banvoa understood my words. The most important thing I can tell her (to me) is that the one person she should never be afraid to talk to - is YOU. A mother should be open to whatever her daughter is trying to express or needs help with. I am so happy to see a relationship like the one you have with Banvoa, and I know that through your work you will inspire other mothers and daughters. I loved Toni's (sp) singing and it brought me to tears. I love Ms. Ursula and Ms. Gwen's advice and I will adhere to their words. I LOVED, LOVED Malane's words, aura, and whole vibe (sp) - she got some POWER! And I sho' will hit up that JeJu Salon! lol In closing, it was BEAUTIFUL. A memory that I will keep with me always...I love you, Marlo.
Tiara

It is not an easy or automatic thing to fully, and deeply appreciate what a gift it is to be alive on this green, rich planet. It is even more difficult to appropriately value the living-giving abilities of women. The media and advertisements are full of images of women as mere sex-objects. But the reality is that femininity is deep, sacred, mysterious. Each woman has to journey with care into a full realization of her value. Banvoa and all in her circle are making that journey.
Barbara

WOW. I sense the power of this gathering from reading your words. And I was really touched by the shedding of your tears in this space of healing. Truly you are setting a solid foundation for Banvoa by helping her to understand that the body is sacred. The violence that we see in the world today is in part due to the lack of understanding of this. Most parents do not know how to teach this and wind up passing their own fears and projections back onto their children. Banvoa is blessed in learning this at a pivotal age.
Blessings Antoinette

Awesome, awesome, awesome. How comforting, how hope-giving it is to know there are still people in the world who honor and respect tradition, the passing on of wisdom, the celebration of youth and all its unfettered hope and dynamism. It DOES take a "village" of souls to carry us, give us strength, a reason to love, a dream to formulate, mold and achieve. The presence of all who were there, whether physically or not reaffirms how spirit seeks spirit and lifts us to the greatest heights the human heart can reach. While I read your description of the day, I was almost moved to tears myself! I feel no lack of maternal love simply because my biological child never got to walk the earth – my children, my parents, my cousins, aunties, and uncles, are anywhere and everywhere that people of the "grand love" gather together and celebrate!

Blessings to each and every one from the Mojave Desert of California, and God's peace and power to all!!
Sandy

Hi Marlo,
This sounds absolutely wonderful!!!!! I am so happy about this glorious event. I agree with Armel that this is an appropriate way to go. I think the parents should collectively offer words and then the fathers should exit and let the women continue. Great idea!
Ayanna

Banvoa is a beautiful young lady. Thank you for sharing this experience!!
Robin

Hi Marlo, finally got to read about what sounds like a moving, enjoyable and particularly important event in many lives. As one far removed from the flowering of youth and even from being around young adolescents, I must say that I found myself wishing that my generation had mothers and aunts and friends like those your daughter has. (NOTE: our mothers, aunts and friends were great, and did what they could at the time) I have been sharing information about this event with young (and not so young) mothers and grandmothers. I do hope you will use your many talents to inform, suggest and persuade others of the importance of what you are doing. Stay well.
Sincerely, Karen

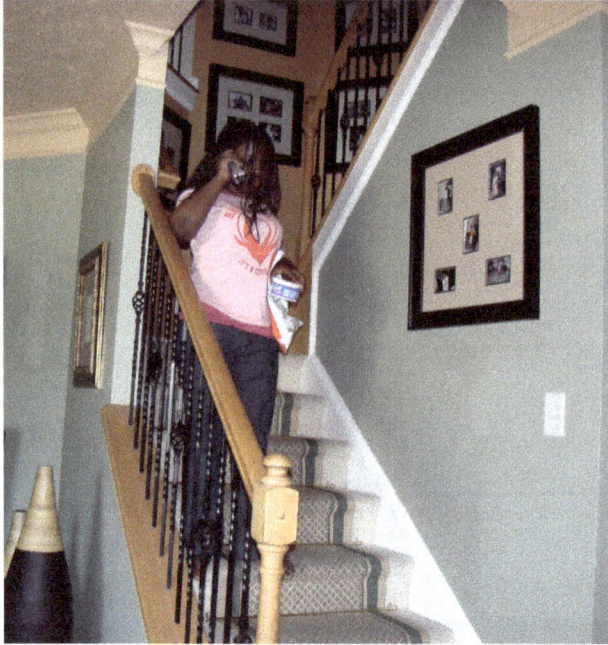

Banvoa calling women in her sacred circle to share entry into womanhood at the start of her period.

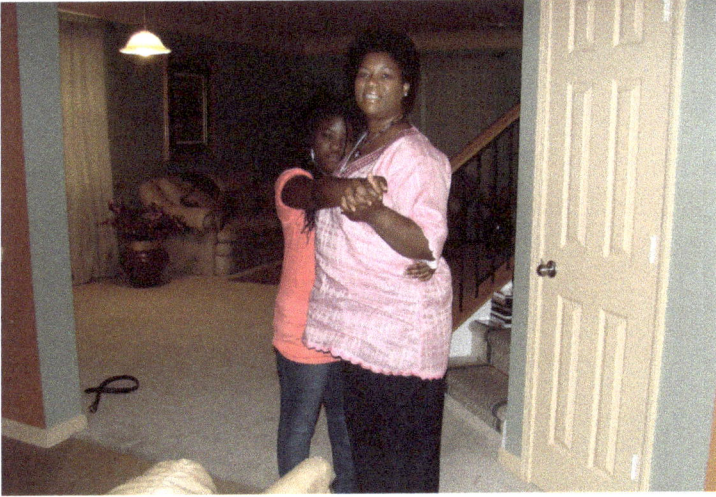

Mother and daughter sharing loving embrace as women.

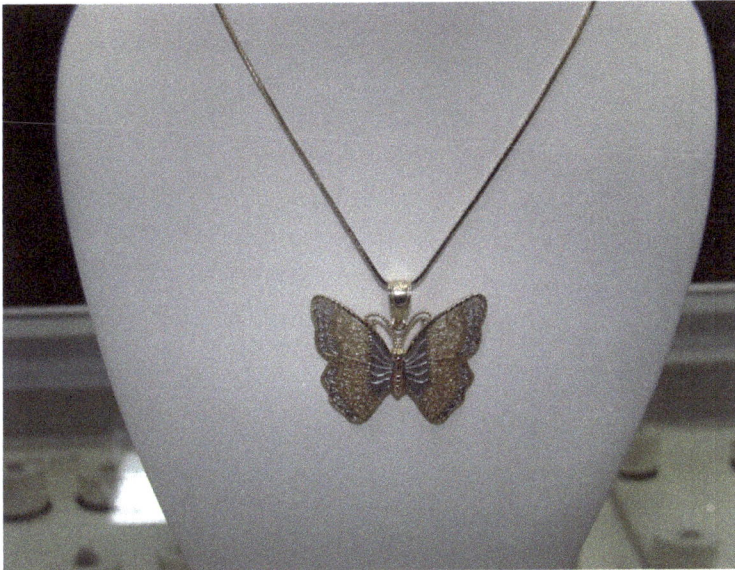

**Butterfly necklace symbolizing transformation
into womanhood.**

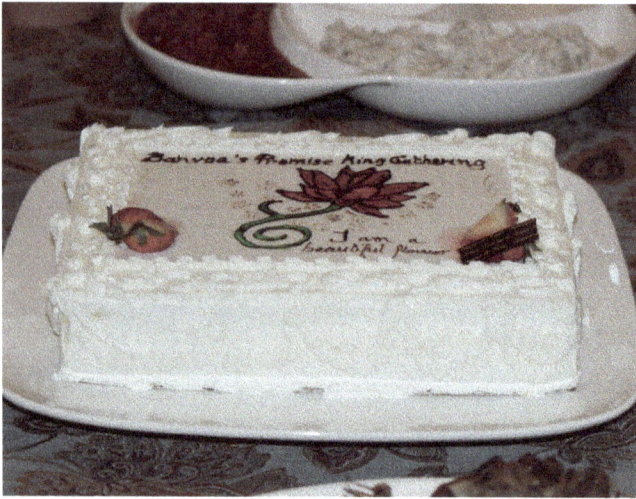

Promise Ring Gathering cake.

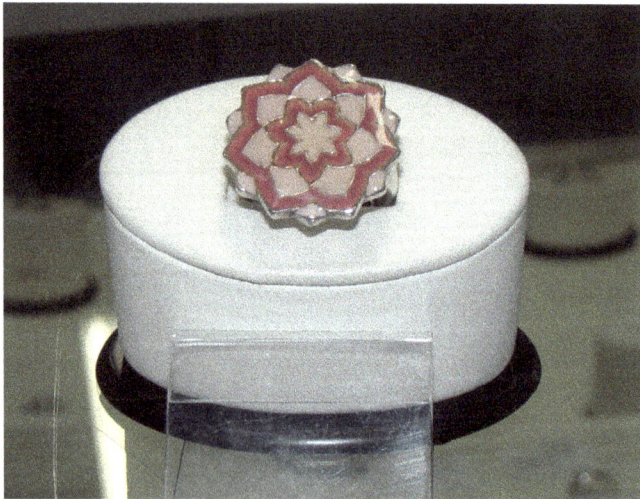

Banvoa's pink lotus promise ring to keep her body sacred through abstinence.

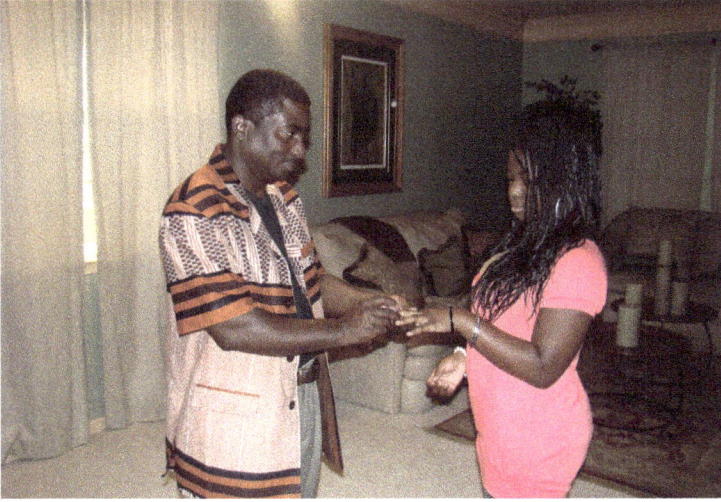

Banvoa receives promise ring from proud Daddy.

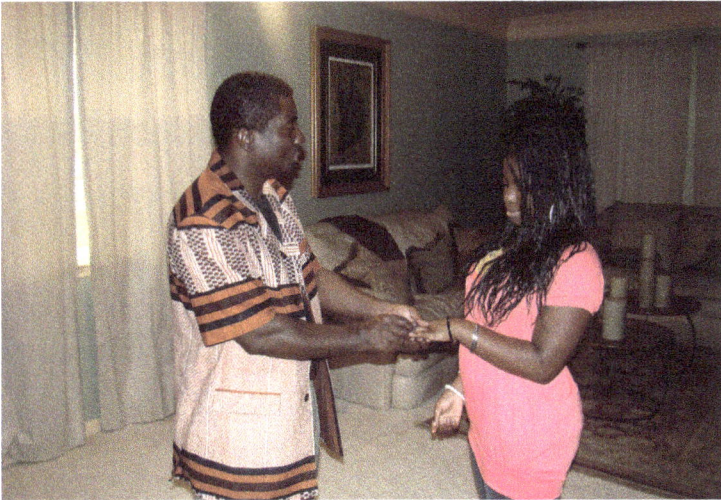

Banvoa receives promise ring and advice.

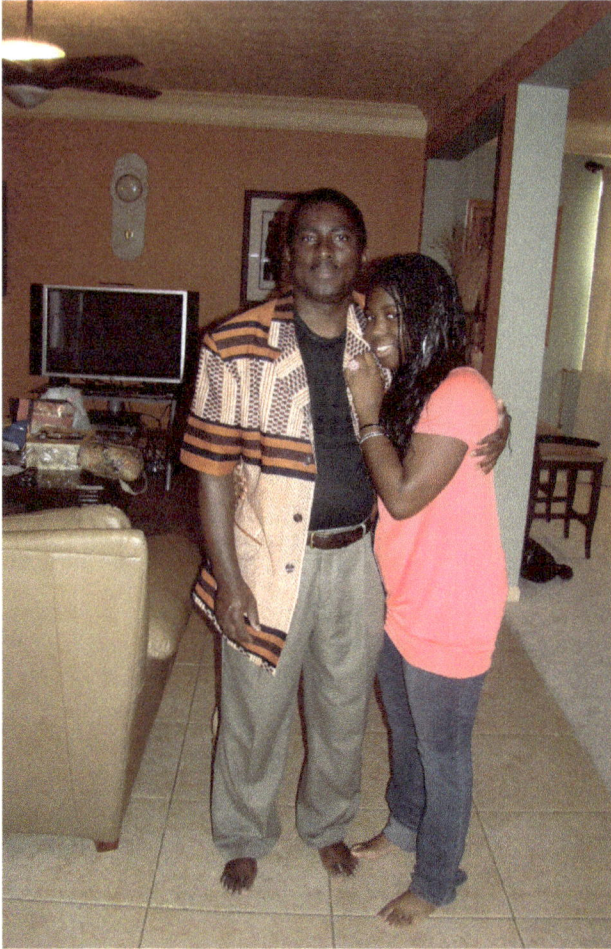

Proud Daddy and his promised daughter.

Conclusion

Dear reader, we have now come to the end of our journey together, as what every flowering girl should know has been shared. Thank you, reader. May all or most of your questions about the basic biology of your body have been answered in this reading because it is for you. Considering basic biology of the body, we began our quest discussing the cycle of life with how many eggs a female has as a baby girl, ovulation, uterine changes, menstruation, cramps, premenstrual changes, and menopause. You now have a reproductive system vocabulary that you may refer to, that will answer some of the most fundamental questions about female and male reproduction; the importance of nutrition for a healthy female and male reproductive system such as, water, vitamins, electrolytes, amino acids, and the 21 essential minerals your mind and body needs; a variety of herbs that support reproductive and immune systems; digestive enzymes; the differences between prebiotics and probiotics. Because you now have a basic understanding of the reproductive system and its nutritional needs for optimal health, information about pregnancy and its three trimesters and how the baby develops month to month is next, and lastly, the most glaring question during pregnancy is: Will the Fetus be Female or Male, which is determined by chromosomes?

Again, thank you for the opportunity to share this work. May the bond between you, your mother, (your guardian, if you don't have a mother) and all of the most important women in your life, your sacred circle of love and care be strengthened. Remember dear reader, you are a lotus, and your body is sacred. May your story be written to be cherished and told to the female generation that comes behind you. As the introduction of "I Am a Beautiful Flower, What Every Flowering Girl Should Know" started with sharing my daughters flowering story that led to having a Flower Party and a year later a Promise Ring Gathering, this is the delight of having the parties:

The Flowering Party encourages the young girl not to be afraid of her menstrual cycle, but to embrace it as a natural phase her body experiences as a part of the reproductive system. The Flowering Party is a comforting moment of sharing and bonding between mother, daughter and other women who cherish and support the woman to be in her growth and maturity—a sacred circle of women who will always be available to her. In representing another opportunity for the young girl to better understand the biology of her body, the Flowering Party helps to build the girl's self-esteem and worth. Such awareness helps to cultivate more meaningful and mutually respectful relationships with boys. It may also assist in helping to curtail the national epidemic of teenage pregnancy by promoting abstinence as a method of birth control.

The Promise Ring Gathering is an extension of the Flowering Party. It is an acknowledgement of the girl continuing to embrace the sacredness of her body. It marks the first year of the abstinent young woman experiencing her menstrual cycle. It is also for the young woman who is recommitting herself to being abstinent. We need our daughters to think with understanding about the consequences of their actions before they make the choice. The Flowering Party and Promise Ring Gathering are intimate times that mindfully nurture and celebrate the femininity of the young girl as she enters womanhood.

A flowering girl who is blossoming as the newest member of an ever-expanding circle of women, who as a part of nature, are a balancing half for continuing life. As with other projects, the Flowering Party and Promise Ring Gathering is just another layer of fabric in a large quilt that is seeking to affirm young girls. Our daughters are beautiful flowers, and we love them. These are two empowering ways to expand their awareness and continue to help them make sound choices regarding their bodies. With the plethora of information, that the I Am a Beautiful Flower book provides, our daughters will know that they are loved and so will you.

.

www.ingramcontent.com/pod-product-compliance
Lightning Source LLC
Chambersburg PA
CBHW052112030426
42335CB00025B/2956